P9-BBU-858

THE 4-Ingredient
DIABETES COOKBOOK

Simple, Quick, and Delicious Recipes Using Just Four Ingredients or Less!

NANCY S. HUGHES

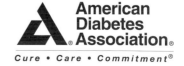

American Diabetes Association.
Cure • Care • Commitment®

Managing Editor, Book Publishing, Abe Ogden; *Acquisitions Editor, Consumer Books,* Robert Anthony; *Editor,* Laurie Guffey; *Production Manager,* Melissa Sprott; *Composition and Cover Design,* pixiedesign llc; *Printer,* Transcontinental Printing.

©2007 by Nancy S. Hughes. All Rights Reserved. No part of this publication may be reproduced or transmitted in any form or by any means, electronic or mechanical, including duplication, recording, or any information storage and retrieval system, without the prior written permission of the American Diabetes Association.

Printed in Canada
3 5 7 9 10 8 6 4

The suggestions and information contained in this publication are generally consistent with the Clinical Practice Recommendations and other policies of the American Diabetes Association, but they do not represent the policy or position of the Association or any of its boards or committees. Reasonable steps have been taken to ensure the accuracy of the information presented. However, the American Diabetes Association cannot ensure the safety or efficacy of any product or service described in this publication. Individuals are advised to consult a physician or other appropriate health care professional before undertaking any diet or exercise program or taking any medication referred to in this publication. Professionals must use and apply their own professional judgment, experience, and training and should not rely solely on the information contained in this publication before prescribing any diet, exercise, or medication. The American Diabetes Association—its officers, directors, employees, volunteers, and members—assumes no responsibility or liability for personal or other injury, loss, or damage that may result from the suggestions or information in this publication.

∞ The paper in this publication meets the requirements of the ANSI Standard Z39.48-1992 (permanence of paper).

ADA titles may be purchased for business or promotional use or for special sales. To purchase more than 50 copies of this book at a discount, or for custom editions of this book with your logo, contact Lee Romano Sequeira, Special Sales & Promotions, at the address below, or at LRomano@diabetes.org or 703-299-2046.

For all other inquiries, please call 1-800-DIABETES.

American Diabetes Association
1701 North Beauregard Street
Alexandria, Virginia 22311

Library of Congress Cataloging-in-Publication Data

Hughes, Nancy S.
    The 4-ingredient diabetes cookbook / Nancy S. Hughes
        p.cm.
    Includes bibliographical references and index.
    ISBN 978-1-58040-278-1 (alk. paper)
  1. Diabetes--Diet therapy--Recipes. I. Title. II. Title: Four ingredient diabetes cookbook.

RC662.H83 2007
641.5'6314--dc22
           2007015971

TO MY HUSBAND, GREG

You've given me inspiration, guidance, and unbelievable support…
with an unshakable sense of humor!

You'll never stop fascinating me.

CONTENTS

ACKNOWLEDGEMENTS

From concocting the initial concept to meeting the final deadline, I can honestly say I couldn't have done it alone...who could or would? There's the shopping, chopping, measuring, cooking, cleaning up, and starting all over again, plus the retyping, rethinking, recalculating, reshaping...and all the stuff in between. Who to thank first?

- my husband, Greg, for putting up with the chaos of the alarm clock going off at 3 A.M., never knowing what he could eat in the refrigerator (because it might be used to develop a recipe), and the dishwasher running constantly;

- my family, Annie, Taft, Will, and Kelly, for taste-testing every single time they'd come in AND out the door;

- my editor, Rob Anthony, for believing in me, getting excited with me, and calmly humoring me when I'd ramble on about the latest developed recipe;

- Robin Brinker and Jess Hendry, for their hard work and high-energy attitude in and out of the kitchen, which helped me keep my own energy level up and the creativity flowing...no matter what time it was;

- and Liz Dixon, for her passion for learning about food and how it works, which took her from long, long hours on her feet in my kitchen to earning a well-deserved scholarship in Food Science at the college of her choice, Auburn University.

See, I told you I couldn't do it alone.

Thanks for being there for me.

Nancy

INTRODUCTION

WHY ONE MORE COOKBOOK?

This book is for people with diabetes—or those who want to eat healthier—but who don't want to live in the kitchen. Inside you'll find 150 delicious recipes, all made with four ingredients or less! (In case you're checking up on me, salt, pepper, water, and cooking spray don't count as ingredients, and I counted the zest and juice of the same fruit as one ingredient.) Some of these recipes even call for three or only two ingredients, and still taste scrumptious. When you stop and think about what this actually means and how it can affect your lifestyle—and your workload—you may never want to cook any other way again. Using fewer ingredients means fewer items in your grocery cart, less time in the grocery line, fewer items to unload and put away when you get home, less time to prepare the dish, and—my personal favorite—fewer pots and pans to clean! You'll actually have time to do... well, anything else you want, because you won't be stuck in the kitchen (or in the grocery store) all of the time.

I consider myself a lazy cook. I'm always looking for that shorter cut, that quicker way, that anything to help me avoid work. But at the same time, I want every bit of effort I do make to count. When my editor and I were discussing the prospect of writing this much-needed book, he looked me straight in the eye and said, "150 recipes, Nancy, you're sure you can create 150 recipes that use only 4 ingredients, meet our nutritional standards, and still taste great?" I knew it would be a challenge—even though I've been developing quick and healthy recipes for over 25 years—but I wanted to introduce a new approach to people whose lives may already be burdened with numbers, counting, and chores. I wanted to show people how to discover that simpler is better, and faster can be more delicious, when every ingredient really counts.

The secret, I found, is not the number of ingredients, but rather the different types of ingredients and the various techniques included in the recipes. For example, by using highly flavored ingredients and convenience foods that contain several ingredients in one product, such as picante sauce or herb blends, I can shorten the ingredient list drastically without compromising on flavor. As for effective techniques, something as simple as searing or reducing ingredients (that is, cooking them down to a more concentrated form over high heat) is an extremely easy, fast way to get intense flavor without adding extra ingredients, fat, or time.

If you keep the meal prep simple but the great flavor's still there, you'll find yourself returning to the same healthy recipes over and over again. That's my whole point in writing this book: to help people with diabetes stay on a healthy track all of the time, bringing them delicious flavors and fresh new ideas that will last them a lifetime. My no-hassle approach is just that…easy and approachable, so that everyone can have the "I can do THAT!" attitude.

And the whole reason I published with the American Diabetes Association is that together, we've done the work for you. You can trust that ALL these recipes are good for you and taste delicious, too. We've given you all the numbers to help you monitor your intake of fat, sodium, and carb. You don't have to worry if the recipes are "okay" for you. You can enjoy great-tasting, quick, and simple meals without the math swirling in your head all of the time…and with a fraction of the work!

KITCHEN TOOLS YOU'LL REALLY USE

Besides the usual pots, pans, cookie sheets, measuring cups, and slotted spoons, there are certain items that make cooking faster and easier…and they're very economical because not only are they inexpensive, they save you time.

- **Fine grater.** This is also known as a microplane. It's great for zesting (that is, grating the peel from a citrus fruit) and finely grating hard cheeses, fresh gingerroot, and even garlic. It's made of stainless steel that has been perforated with sharp-edged, small holes. Buy the variety that is made of stainless steel, rather than tin, so it won't rust. Also, choose the style that has a rubber handle or grip at the top for better control. A fine grater makes grating easy and effortless!

- **Garlic press.** This tool is used to press a garlic clove through tiny holes, which extracts both the pulp and the juice. I think so much more garlic flavor is released using a garlic press than with chopping, because pressing produces a finer texture and the oils and flavors are not absorbed into the cutting board. You can place a small or medium clove in the garlic press without peeling it, then press down. The meat of the garlic comes through, leaving behind the peel! Larger cloves of garlic need to be halved first. (And here's a bizarre garlic tip for you: to neutralize the garlic aroma on your fingertips, wash your hands, then run your fingertips over any chrome you may have, such as your faucet or towel bar. The aroma magically disappears! You have to try this and see for yourself.)

- **Hand-held wooden reamer.** This is used for juicing citrus fruits, such as lemons, limes, and oranges. It is a ridged, teardrop-shaped tool with a handle. Simply cut the fruit in half crosswise and press it into the point of the reamer. Twist the reamer back and forth to extract the juices. You get so much more juice out of the fruit than you could by simply squeezing it with your hands.

- **Gravy or fat separator.** This removes grease from hot cooking liquid. It is a small, clear pitcher made of glass or heatproof plastic. You pour the hot liquid into the pitcher and allow it to stand for 2 to 3 minutes, and the fat will rise to the top. The pitcher is designed so that the liquid can be poured out, leaving the grease behind. (See page 91 for another great fat separator tip.)

- **Small fine-mesh sieve.** This helps you strain or deseed raspberries or anything with small bits or pieces that need to be removed. Use it for sifting small amounts of powdered sugar evenly over cakes and cookies, too.

- **Silicone spatulas.** These are basically rubber spatulas that can stand the heat. Use them with nonstick skillets and saucepans to scrape their bottoms and sides, collecting all of the concentrated flavors that accumulate there while cooking. They are also gentler on ingredients when stirring and tossing and prevent the ingredients from breaking down too much. Buy several different sizes to keep on hand.

- **Metal or plastic ruler.** Yep, I'm not kidding. Use one to accurately measure ingredients that need to be cut into 1-inch cubes, 1/2-inch wedges, or 2-inch strips. You'll soon learn how to do this without measuring, and your cooking results will be more successful if your same-sized ingredients cook evenly.

- **Kitchen scale.** The scales in the produce aisles aren't always accurate, and sometimes it's hard to divide out the correct amount of meat and seafood you need for any given recipe. The best way to be accurate is to weigh it on your own scales. Buy the variety with a removable tray so it can go in the dishwasher or be cleaned easily. You'll be surprised how often you use it.

- **Vegetable peeler with a rubber handle.** You may already have your favorite kind of vegetable peeler, but I love this variety because, more times than not, I have wet hands when working in the kitchen, and the rubber handle keeps them from slipping—which makes it a lot faster to get the job done. To make the job go even faster, peel the vegetables under running water. The peeling slips away into the garbage disposal as you peel. There's another step saved!

- **Digital timer.** You can find this in discount stores for practically nothing. To me, they are more accurate than the wind-up variety. Whether you're timing something for 1 minute or 1 hour, just set it for the time you want and know it will be accurate. I time everything, from preheating a skillet, to reducing a 1-minute sauce, to letting a cooked cut of meat stand before slicing. It helps me keep from overheating or underheating a skillet, burning a sauce, and basically ruining a lot of recipes!

- **Mini muffin tins.** These are a fraction of the standard size, but you will feel more satisfied if you bake your muffins and quick breads in them, because you can have more than one! They're nice to serve when entertaining, too. Try making mini quiches with them—great for a brunch buffet table.

- **Paper towels.** Yes, a paper towel can be a very functional tool, beyond drying your hands and cleaning up spills. Use a damp paper towel to wipe mushrooms clean, to pat chicken or fish dry before cooking, to aid in removing the skin from chicken (it provides the traction needed), and—my personal favorite—when you put a couple of damp paper towels under a cutting board, they keep the cutting board in place instead of slipping and sliding around!

PULL, PREP, AND PREHEAT

Before you actually start to cook a recipe, you can do a few things to make the process go even more smoothly.

- **Pull the ingredients.** This sounds obvious, but you'd be surprised how much faster you can cook if you pull everything you need out of the pantry and fridge and line it up on the counter before you start.

- **Prep the ingredients.** Then, start prepping everything you need according to the ingredient list. Have all items prepped before you start following the recipe directions. For example, if the ingredient reads, "1/2 cup chopped onion" or "1 pound boneless sirloin steak, trimmed of fat or cut into 1-inch cubes," have that done before you start the first step. Most of my recipes cook so quickly, you really don't have enough time to chop the onion while the steak cubes are browning.

- **Preheat the skillet.** When a recipe calls for heating the skillet "until hot" before adding ingredients, how can you tell if it's hot enough? An electric range takes about 2 minutes to properly heat a pan. Set your new digital timer so you don't overheat the pan.

Or use the time-honored "pancake test:" sprinkle a few drops of water in the pan. If they "dance" or bounce vigorously, the pan's hot!

MAKE THE MOST OF ALL YOUR MEALS

BREAKFAST

Cereal. Toast. Cereal. Toast. It can get pretty monotonous. Get out of your rut! Take a new approach toward the breakfast meal and what it has to offer.

With our multi-tasking day and night, why not set the breakfast meal to multi-tasking, too? Serve these tasty recipes not only for breakfast, but also for lunch, midday snack, dinner, and even dessert.

Or take a look in the other chapters, such as Beverages or Snacks, and see what would work for a breakfast item. Just choose the recipes to fit your inclinations, while keeping track of your carb intake. I designed these recipes to be versatile enough to fit into other parts of your day as well, giving you even more choices for each meal.

Breakfast Tricks, Tips, and Timesavers

- **Bake a batch.** Muffins or quick breads are perfect for breakfast for one day and a snack or dessert the next. Then freeze the rest in small baggies and pull them out when you need them.

- **Breakfast power drinks.** You can make the beverage recipes in this chapter in just a few minutes, making them great additions to your "on the run" meal or "computer" lunch. Since you need power all day, why not feel as though you're having a treat while you're at it?

- **Double-time your meals.** Make a batch of breakfast-grilled sandwiches, have one for breakfast, and refrigerate the rest. Pop one into the microwave at work or home the next day for a quick "already-made" lunch.

- **Add a veggie or salad.** For dinner, all you need is to steam a few vegetables and toss a fruit salad to transform an omelet or frittata into a fast-fixing dinner option.

- **Reverse it.** Make a fruit drink from the Beverage chapter for breakfast. A fruit drink has fruit juices, fruit, and sometimes yogurt in it…make one a fun and easy part of your breakfast! Or how about using the skillet-grilled fruit in the Fruit Sides chapter to serve alongside your turkey sausage

or Canadian bacon in the morning. It's easy to expand your menu once you start thinking out of the breakfast box.

SNACKS

Portion control is key with snacks and appetizers! It's easier to keep a handle on things when you're in your own home, but when you're at a family gathering or attending a big event, the array of foods spread out before you can be a bit mind boggling. Two things you can do to make it easy on yourself: have a light snack before you go, and don't socialize too close to the buffet table. The light snack will help in curbing your appetite, so you won't be starving when you get there. Keeping your conversations away from the table will prevent you from mindlessly munching while you're visiting. Fix a small plate and move to another area to focus in on your friends, old and new, and have some fun!

Snack Tricks, Tips, and Timesavers

- **Crunch without crackers.** Take a nice break from serving crackers or chips with dip or spreads—try crostini instead. Crostini is a fancy name for little toasted and cooled bread slices. Using baguette bread (the skinny loaf) is your best bet—simply slice, bake briefly, and cool. It's much cheaper than those expensive crackers and chips, too!

- **Spread it out.** Stretch those strong-flavored cheeses as far as they can go by combining a small amount of them with fat-free cream cheese or sour cream. Then add to dips or spreads.

- **Accent the cheese.** Add fresh herbs, such as basil or cilantro, to seasoned light cheese spreads, fat-free cream cheese, or fat-free sour cream, to give tons of flavor in every bite.

- **Small bites need heat.** Add a touch of heat, whether it's with dried pepper flakes, cayenne pepper, chipotle chilis, jalapeño peppers, or hot pepper sauce. The heat intensifies the other flavors in the dish—but remember, a little goes a long way!

- **Fresh is best.** When making fresh salsas, whether they're fruit- or vegetable-based, it's best to serve them within a couple of hours after tossing the ingredients together...otherwise they tend to lose those peak, distinct flavors and become more mellow and blended.

SALADS

There's tossed salads, arranged salads, fruit salads, vegetable-based salads, pasta salads, main dish salads, and potato salads. Use your imagination when making salads—go beyond the bag of greens and a bottle of salad dressing. They're okay in a pinch, but there's a lot more you can do with a salad with little effort and very little fat.

Salad Tricks, Tips, and Timesavers

- **Less dressing, more flavor.** Hold off on some of that dressing and add small amounts of flavorful ingredients instead, such as feta or Parmesan cheese, artichoke hearts, olives, lean ham or turkey pepperoni, and, of course, fresh herbs.

- **Think small tomatoes.** You can always rely on those little sweet grape tomatoes for that year-round, peak-season flavor. They're packed with concentrated flavors that burst with sweetness. Cut them in half to make the flavors (and your dollar) go twice as far!

- **Cut the mayo.** But hang onto flavor and texture.
  - Replace part of the mayonnaise with fat-free sour cream.

- Use a reduced-fat creamy salad dressing, such as Ranch, for pasta- and potato-based salads. Be sure to incorporate other highly flavored ingredients, such as onion or green peppers, to balance flavor and texture.

- Add low-fat buttermilk to your mayo-based salad dressings. It adds thickness and gives a lift to the other ingredient flavors while tying everything together.

- **Toast those nuts.** Even if it's just 2 tablespoons of nuts, the nutty flavor will travel so much further if you toast them…and it takes just 2 minutes in a hot skillet.

- **Ditch the seeds.** Tomatoes and cucumbers are often seeded in recipes. It's an important step—don't skip it. Removing the seeds prevents the dish from getting too much liquid in it and diluting the other flavors.

  - There are two ways to seed a tomato. First, halve the tomato crosswise (that's parallel to the stem portion of the tomato) and squeeze the juices and seeds out; or halve the tomato the same way, then place your clean fingertips in the seed pockets. The juices and seeds will rise to the surface and you can push them out.

  - To seed a cucumber, cut it in half lengthwise, and run the tip of a teaspoon down the center to scrape the seeds out easily.

- **Shake and serve.** Bottled in-gredients, particularly soy sauce, Worcestershire sauce, and, of course, salad dressings, really do need to be shaken before using. I know that sounds a bit elementary, but it does make a big difference.

SOUPS

Soup makes a perfect partner for salads and sandwiches. It can bring much-needed comfort after a hard day, or act as a special first course when you're entertaining. But did you know that soup can be loaded with sodium, bank-rupt of nutrition, and exploding with fat and carb? Be careful when you're in a restaurant or grabbing a couple of cans from your grocer's shelves. Ask questions, read labels, and think twice before you order. The soups in this book are worry-free and packed with flavor and nutrition…all the good things that should be connected with the soup you eat!

Soup Tricks, Tips, and Timesavers

- **Stock up.** Keep a variety of frozen vegetables and vegetable combinations stored away to make a quick soup anytime you feel like it. One of my favorite quick veggie items to add to soups is the pepper stir-fry, which contains multicolored pepper strips and onion. It's so versatile, and there's no chopping needed—that's the good part! Keep in mind, though, that the onions in the stir-fry take longer to cook than other vegetables, about 20 minutes.

- **Thaw frozen vegetables quickly.** Place them in a colander and run under cold water 20 to 30 seconds, then shake off excess liquid before continuing with the recipe.

- **Keep those veggies coming.** Keep a resealable quart- or gallon-sized freezer bag in your freezer. Every time you have a few leftover veggies, toss them into the bag—in no time, you'll have enough to make soup! Keep a can of stewed tomatoes and some chicken broth on hand to make soup any time you feel like some.

- **Rinse canned beans.** To remove the thick liquid and some of the sodium, place the beans in a colander, run under cold water, and shake off excess liquid before continuing with the recipe.

- **Make it thick.** No need to add flour or cornstarch. Just use a hand mixer to puree 1 to 1 1/2 cups of the soup, or use a blender and puree until smooth, then return the thick mixture to the saucepot. (It's very important to hold the blender lid down tightly before you turn it on, or your soup will fly everywhere!)

- **Make it fresh.** If you want to add a bit of fresh flavor to your soup, serve it topped with a sprinkling of fresh parsley, green onion, or any fresh herb that is already in the soup.

- **Bring out the cheese.** Reserve a tablespoon or two of the cheese that's supposed to go into the soup and sprinkle it on top at serving time. That enhances a soup's cheesy flavor without increasing calories or fat.

- **Heat it up.** Add some spicy heat in the form of dried red pepper flakes or a little hot pepper sauce just before serving—your soups will taste fuller and more substantial. A little heat goes a long way, so be sure to start with a tiny bit—you can always add more!

MAIN DISHES

Seasonings play a very important part in main dishes. It's important how and when you use them. To get the most flavor from your meats and casseroles, sometimes you need to season before you start to cook, and other times, after. Check the tips below for some great seasoning ideas.

Main Dish Tricks, Tips, and Timesavers

- **Season with the skin on.** Season a chicken or turkey that will be cooked with the skin on by lifting up the skin and rubbing the seasonings between the meat and the skin. Then roast the bird. The seasonings will penetrate into the meat of the bird rather than get lost in the skin that is discarded.

- **Check the label.** Some brands of turkey breast and pork tenderloin have broth or solution added, which means added sodium. Be sure to read the package labels, and if the turkey or pork does contain broth or solution, don't add more salt when cooking it.

- **Use coffee granules.** If you haven't tried using coffee to intensify the hearty flavor of beef, you'll be amazed! Just add 1/2 cup of strong coffee to the roasting pan and pop it in the oven. Or use instant coffee granules dissolved in water. And you don't need to heat the liquid first—the granules dissolve in either hot or cold liquid. Just be sure to stir them well.

- **Deepen the color.** To give a deeper brown appearance to pork, beef, poultry, or fish, dust with a small amount of paprika or chili powder before cooking. Just a light sprinkle will give more color than flavor.

- **Crush those herbs.** Dried herbs take a longer time to release their flavors than fresh or ground varieties, so crush the dried herb leaves between your fingertips before adding them to the dish. Fresh herb flavors are strong, but they fade quickly if cooked for a long time.

- **Using citrus zest and juice.** When a recipe calls for both the zest and juice of a lemon, lime, or orange, always grate the piece of fruit first before squeezing the juice out. It's easier to grate when the fruit is full and firm. Grate only the colorful part of the fruit, not the white pith underneath— that gives the dish a bitter taste.

Main Dish Tricks, Tips, and Timesavers After You Start Cooking

- **Add ground spices.** If you need a stronger, more intense flavor in a dish, add ground spices after cooking. You just need a small amount, and the flavor doesn't break down while cooking.

- **Use a smidgen of sugar.** Add small amounts (1/2 to 1 teaspoon) to stews and skillet dishes. It doesn't add sweetness to the dish, but aids in cutting the acidity of the other ingredients and acts to blend the flavors together.

- **A so-simple sauce.** Reduction is a fancy word for boiling down the liquid in a dish quickly to leave a deeply flavored, intense sauce. This is my favorite cooking trick. Simply add water, broth, or wine to the skillet after sautéing other ingredients. The liquid will absorb the concentrated seasonings that build up in the skillet during the cooking process, then boil down in 1 or 2 minutes to create a quick, highly flavored sauce.

- **Last-minute flavors.** Add the following ingredients to your dishes once they have been removed from the heat. These can also be added to cold entrees at serving time.

- Extracts, such as vanilla and almond extract
- Grated citrus rind and gingerroot
- Flavored oils, such as extra virgin olive oil and sesame oil
- Toasted nuts

STARCHY SIDES

Most nutrition experts will agree that all forms of carb can be okay if you eat them in moderation. But if you ask me, starchy sides are one of the hardest food categories to control. The carb in them can creep up on you if you're not careful. By choosing the right starchy sides and using some of the tricks below, though, you can enjoy them and feel like you've had a large portion without going overboard.

Starchy Side Tricks, Tips, and Timesavers

- **Bulk it up.** Add low-carb vegetables and fruits to a starchy dish to add volume, giving you the feeling that you're eating more than you actually are. This not only adds character to a humdrum side dish, but sneaks in extra vitamins as well. For example, bulk up pasta by tossing in fresh or frozen veggies during the last few minutes of cooking.

- **Break it in thirds.** When using spaghetti noodles as a side, break them in thirds so they are easier to serve and combine better with the vegetables in the dish.

- **Hollow it out.** Heat French bread in the oven, then hollow out the center and use the outer portion for crunchy sandwiches. Save the insides for bread crumbs or croutons—and save some calories, too.

- **Serve it thin.** Instead of a huge hunk of French bread with dinner, bake thin slices of French bread, let them cool slightly, and rub a halved garlic clove lightly over each piece. The larger number of smaller pieces, the delicious crunchiness, and the rich garlic taste will satisfy you well before you eat too much.

- **Sub in some cauliflower.** Cut the amount of potatoes used in your favorite soup recipe by half and substitute with an equal amount of cauliflower. Cauliflower provides great potato-like texture and appearance with much less carb. Try serving mashed cauliflower instead of potatoes.

VEGETABLE SIDES

Night after night of boiled frozen veggies, or heated canned ones, can get really tiresome. The recipes here let you see how easy, interesting, and sensational veggie and fruit sides can be. By preparing them in a variety of ways—roasted, steamed, stuffed, mixed with other vegetables, skillet-grilled, and more—you'll look at vegetable sides in a different light…and find some new favorites.

Vegetable Tricks, Tips, and Timesavers

- **Line it with foil.** When roasting vegetables, always line the baking sheet with foil to protect the baking sheet surface and give you easy clean-up.

- **Maximize your buttery taste.** To get the most concentrated "butter" flavors from light margarine—whether you boil, steam, or roast the veggies— add it after cooking, not during. And don't worry about melting light margarine first—just place it directly on the veggies and let their heat melt it. The flavor of light margarine is so much better that way.

- **The right cut.** How you cut a vegetable is important, so be sure to follow the recipe's instructions. Veggie cut affects the evenness of cooking, cooking time, and recipe presentation, so follow directions to be successful!

DESSERTS

Here is where choosing the right carb can really make the most difference. By using lower-fat versions of cream cheese, ice cream, and yogurt; by including plenty of fresh fruits, berries, and melon; and by choosing truly delicious recipes to prepare, you'll end up with a scrumptious, decent-sized dessert on your plate—and you'll be satisfied without wanting to overindulge. These recipes and the tricks below help you have the sweet stuff—the cakes, pies, parfaits, and ice-cream desserts—without going out of bounds.

Dessert Tricks, Tips, and Timesavers

- **Have your snack cake and eat it, too.** You can make your own snack cakes quickly and easily from boxed cake mixes. Simply add fruit—any fruit you like, either mashed or the jarred baby food version—instead of oil and cook the cake a few minutes less. To see if your snack cake is done, test it with a wooden toothpick. When the toothpick comes out almost clean, the cake's done. It will continue to cook while cooling and will stay moist.

- **Stretch your snack cake.** Bake the snack cake batter in mini muffin tins but cook them a few minutes less. These little cakes are great for a midmorning snack or a brown bag lunch.

- **Rev up the chocolate flavor.** Add a bit of instant coffee granules to chocolate cake mixes and brownie mixes for a deeper chocolaty flavor.

- **Sweeten fruit-based desserts.** Use all-fruit spreads instead of sugar. Heat the fruit spread briefly in the microwave to melt it slightly, and then toss it with your favorite fruit or add it to your favorite recipe.

- **Make a mini pie.** Make individual tarts using refrigerated piecrust, cutting rounds with a biscuit cutter and baking in muffin tins. Serve them with a spoonful of sugar-free whipped topping and overflowing with fresh fruit.

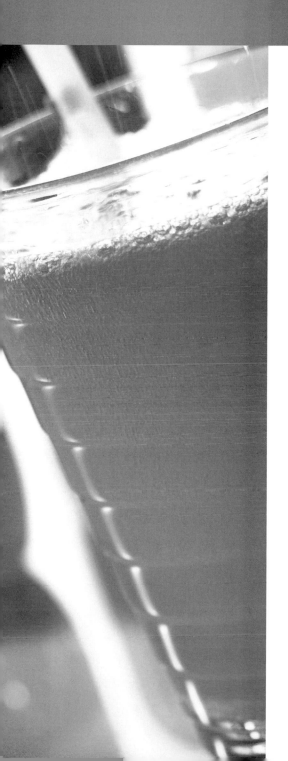

BEVERAGES

PINEAPPLE–APRICOT FIZZ

Serves 4/Serving size: 1 cup

PREP TIME: 5 MINUTES

2 cups cold pineapple juice
(or pineapple, orange, and banana juice blend)

1 cup cold apricot nectar

1 cup diet ginger ale

1 Combine the juice and nectar in a pitcher and stir. Pour into 4 tall glasses with ice.

2 Add 1/4 cup ginger ale to each serving and stir gently to blend. Serve immediately.

COOK'S TIP

Be sure to shake the nectar well before you measure! For more fizz, add 1/4 cup additional ginger ale to each serving.

EXCHANGES

2 Fruit

Calories 105
  Calories from Fat 0

Total Fat 0 g
  Saturated Fat 0 g

Cholesterol 0 mg

Sodium 14 mg

Total Carbohydrate 26 g
  Dietary Fiber 1 g
  Sugars 22 g

Protein 1 g

CAPPUCCINO CHILLER

Serves 4/Serving size: 1/2 cup

PREP TIME: 5 MINUTES

2 cups fat-free, sugar-free vanilla ice cream

1 cup water

1 tablespoon instant coffee granules

4 ice cubes or 1/2 cup coarsely crushed ice

1 Place all ingredients in a blender and blend until smooth.

2 Sweeten to taste with pourable sugar substitute.

COOK'S TIP

This recipe easily doubles, but make it in two batches for easier blending.

EXCHANGES

1 1/2 Carbohydrate

Calories 82
  Calories from Fat 0
Total Fat 0 g
  Saturated Fat 0 g
Cholesterol 4 mg
Sodium 74 mg
Total Carbohydrate 20 g
  Dietary Fiber 5 g
  Sugars 5 g
Protein 4 g

TROPICAL STRAWBERRY CREAM

Serves 3/Serving size: 1 cup

PREP TIME: 4 MINUTES

1 cup fat-free, artificially sweetened, vanilla-flavored yogurt

1 1/4 cups whole strawberries, stems removed

1/2 ripe medium banana

6-ounce can pineapple juice

1. Place all ingredients in a blender and blend until smooth.

COOK'S TIP

You can make this recipe up to 24 hours before serving.

EXCHANGES

1 Fruit
1/2 Fat-Free Milk

Calories 98
  Calories from Fat 0

Total Fat 0 g
  Saturated Fat 0 g

Cholesterol 2 mg

Sodium 41 mg

Total Carbohydrate 22 g
  Dietary Fiber 2 g
  Sugars 16 g

Protein 3 g

COOK'S TIP

For a stronger ginger flavor, cover the tea with plastic wrap and refrigerate overnight or at least 8 hours.

EXCHANGES

Free Food

Calories 13
  Calories from Fat 0

Total Fat 0 g
  Saturated Fat 0 g

Cholesterol 0 mg

Sodium 26 mg

Total Carbohydrate 3 g
  Dietary Fiber 0 g
  Sugars 3 g

Protein 0 g

CRANBERRY-SPLASHED GINGER TEA

Serves 4/Serving size: 1 cup

PREP TIME: 5 MINUTES
STAND TIME: 30 MINUTES

3 cups water

2 tea bags

Four 2-inch long gingerroot pieces, peeled

1 cup artificially sweetened cranberry juice cocktail

2–3 tablespoons pourable sugar substitute

1 Bring the water to a boil in a medium saucepan over high heat. Remove from the heat, add tea bags and gingerroot, and steep for 2 minutes.

2 Remove the tea bags. Let the gingerroot and tea stand for 30 minutes.

3 Pour the tea and gingerroot into a small pitcher, add the juice and sugar substitute, and stir until blended. Refrigerate until needed, then remove ginger and serve over ice.

SWEET CITRUS COOLER

Serves 4/Serving size: 3/4 cup

PREP TIME: 5 MINUTES

1 1/2 cups water
1 cup white grape juice
3–4 tablespoons lemon juice
3–4 tablespoons lime juice
3 tablespoons pourable sugar substitute

1 Combine all ingredients in a small pitcher and stir until well blended.

2 Refrigerate until needed.

COOK'S TIP

Use fresh lemon and lime juice for peak flavors. One medium lemon or lime yields about 2 tablespoons of juice.

EXCHANGES
1 Fruit

Calories 49
  Calories from Fat 0

Total Fat 0 g
  Saturated Fat 0 g

Cholesterol 0 mg

Sodium 11 mg

Total Carbohydrate 12 g
  Dietary Fiber 0 g
  Sugars 11 g

Protein 0 g

MOCHA POWER PICK-UP

Serves 6/Serving size: 1/2 cup

PREP TIME: 4 MINUTES

2 cups fat-free half-and-half

2 packets (0.53 ounces each) sugar-free hot cocoa mix

2 tablespoons reduced-fat peanut butter

1/2–1 teaspoon instant coffee granules

1/2 cup ice cubes (optional)

1. Place all ingredients in a blender and blend until smooth.

EXCHANGES

1 Carbohydrate
1/2 Fat

Calories 99
   Calories from Fat 30

Total Fat 3 g
   Saturated Fat 1 g

Cholesterol 4 mg

Sodium 164 mg

Total Carbohydrate 13 g
   Dietary Fiber 1 g
   Sugars 7 g

Protein 4 g

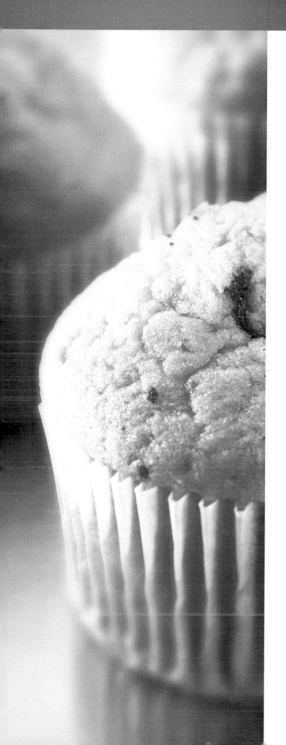

BREAKFAST

GOOD MORNING POWER PARFAIT

Serves 4/Serving size: 1 parfait

PREP TIME: 5 MINUTES

1 ripe medium banana

2 cups fat-free, artificially sweetened, vanilla-flavored yogurt (divided use)

1 teaspoon ground cinnamon (optional)

2 1/2 cups whole strawberries, quartered

1/2 cup grape-nut-style cereal, preferably with raisins and almonds

1 Add the banana, 1 cup yogurt, and cinnamon (if using) to a blender and blend until smooth. Pour into 4 wine or parfait glasses.

2 Top each parfait with a rounded cup of strawberries, 1/4 cup yogurt, and 2 tablespoons cereal.

COOK'S TIP

This parfait's a great way to start your day— it's packed with Vitamin C and fiber!

EXCHANGES

1 Starch
1/2 Fruit
1/2 Fat-Free Milk

Calories 142
  Calories from Fat 8

Total Fat 1 g
  Saturated Fat 0 g

Cholesterol 3 mg

Sodium 113 mg

Total Carbohydrate 30 g
  Dietary Fiber 4 g
  Sugars 15 g

Protein 6 g

BUSY DAY BREAKFAST BURRITO

Serves 4/Serving size: 1 burrito

PREP TIME: 5 MINUTES
COOK TIME: 3 MINUTES

1 1/2 cups egg substitute

4 6-inch flour tortillas

1/4 cup picante sauce

1/2 cup shredded, reduced-fat, sharp cheddar cheese

1 Place a small nonstick skillet over medium heat until hot. Coat the skillet with nonstick cooking spray, add egg substitute, and cook, without stirring, until egg mixture begins to set on bottom, about 1 minute.

2 Draw a spatula across the bottom of pan to form large curds. Continue cooking until egg mixture is thick but still moist; do not stir constantly.

3 Place the tortillas on a microwave-safe plate and microwave on HIGH for 15 seconds or until heated. Top each with equal amounts of the egg mixture.

4 Spoon 1 tablespoon salsa evenly over the egg on each tortilla, sprinkle with 2 tablespoons cheese, and roll up.

COOK'S TIP

Use extra-sharp cheddar cheese for a more intense cheese flavor. In general, this is a great way to stretch the cheese flavor in recipes without adding fat or calories.

EXCHANGES

1 1/2 Starch
1 Lean Meat
1/2 Fat

Calories 203
  Calories from Fat 53

Total Fat 6 g
  Saturated Fat 2 g

Cholesterol 10 mg

Sodium 643 mg

Total Carbohydrate 21 g
  Dietary Fiber 1 g
  Sugars 2 g

Protein 16 g

ENGLISH MUFFIN MELTS

Serves 8/Serving size: 1 melt

PREP TIME: 12 MINUTES
COOK TIME: 3 MINUTES

4 whole wheat English muffins, cut in half
2 tablespoons reduced-fat mayonnaise
3 ounces sliced reduced-fat Swiss cheese, torn in small pieces
4 ounces oven-roasted deli turkey, finely chopped

1   Preheat the broiler.

2   Arrange the muffin halves on a baking sheet and place under the broiler for 1–2 minutes or until lightly toasted. Remove from broiler and spread 3/4 teaspoon mayonnaise over each muffin half.

3   Arrange the cheese pieces evenly on each muffin half and top with the turkey.

4   Return to the broiler and cook 3 minutes, or until the turkey is just beginning to turn golden and the cheese has melted.

COOK'S TIP

Be sure to arrange the items in the order suggested—the cheese has a creamier texture when you place it on top of the mayonnaise.

EXCHANGES
1 Starch
1/2 Fat

Calories 117
    Calories from Fat 33
Total Fat 4 g
    Saturated Fat 1 g
Cholesterol 11 mg
Sodium 309 mg
Total Carbohydrate 13 g
    Dietary Fiber 2 g
    Sugars 2 g
Protein 9 g

SWEET ONION FRITTATA WITH HAM

Serves 4/Serving size: 1/4 recipe

PREP TIME: 15 MINUTES
COOK TIME: 8 MINUTES
STAND TIME: 3 MINUTES

4 ounces extra lean, low-sodium ham slices, chopped

1 cup thinly sliced Vidalia onion

1 1/2 cups egg substitute

1/2 cup shredded, reduced-fat, sharp cheddar cheese

1 Place a medium nonstick skillet over medium-high heat until hot. Coat the skillet with nonstick cooking spray, add ham, and cook until beginning to lightly brown, about 2–3 minutes, stirring frequently. Remove from skillet and set aside on separate plate.

2 Reduce the heat to medium, coat the skillet with nonstick cooking spray, add onions, and cook 4 minutes or until beginning to turn golden, stirring frequently.

3 Reduce the heat to medium low, add ham to the onions, and cook 1 minute (this allows the flavors to blend and the skillet to cool slightly before the eggs are added). Pour egg substitute evenly over all, cover, and cook 8 minutes or until puffy and set.

4 Remove the skillet from the heat, sprinkle cheese evenly over all, cover, and let stand 3 minutes to melt the cheese and develop flavors.

COOK'S TIP

If Vidalia onions are not available, use any other sweet variety, such as Texas Sweet.

EXCHANGES

1 Vegetable
2 Lean Meat

Calories 132
  Calories from Fat 32

Total Fat 4 g
  Saturated Fat 2 g

Cholesterol 23 mg

Sodium 519 mg

Total Carbohydrate 7 g
  Dietary Fiber 1 g
  Sugars 4 g

Protein 18 g

CHEESY MUSHROOM OMELET

Serves 2/Serving size: 1/2 omelet

PREP TIME: 4 MINUTES
COOK TIME: 6 MINUTES

6 ounces sliced mushrooms

1/8 teaspoon salt

1/8 teaspoon black pepper

1/3 cup finely chopped green onion (green and white parts)

1 cup egg substitute

1 ounce crumbled bleu cheese (about 1/4 cup)
or 1/4 cup shredded, reduced-fat, sharp cheddar cheese

1 Place a small skillet over medium-high heat until hot. Coat with nonstick cooking spray and add mushrooms, salt, and pepper. Coat the mushrooms with nonstick cooking spray and cook 4 minutes or until soft, stirring frequently.

2 Add the onions and cook 1 minute longer. Set the pan aside.

3 Place another small skillet over medium heat until hot. Coat with nonstick cooking spray and add the egg substitute. Cook 1 minute without stirring. Using a rubber spatula, lift up the edges to allow the uncooked portion to run under. Cook 1–2 minutes longer or until eggs are almost set and beginning to puff up slightly.

4 Spoon the mushroom mixture on one half of the omelet, sprinkle the cheese evenly over the mushrooms, and gently fold over. Cut in half to serve.

COOK'S TIP

To double this recipe, cook all of the mushrooms and onions and set them aside. Then make 2 omelets, topping each with half of the mushroom mixture and the cheese. Serve 4 people one omelet half.

EXCHANGES

2 Vegetable
2 Lean Meat

Calories 137
  Calories from Fat 40
Total Fat 4 g
  Saturated Fat 25 g
Cholesterol 11 mg
Sodium 585 mg
Total Carbohydrate 8 g
  Dietary Fiber 1 g
  Sugars 3 g
Protein 17 g

BREAKFAST GRILLED SWISS CHEESE AND RYE

Serves 2/Serving size: 1 sandwich

PREP TIME: 4 MINUTES
COOK TIME: 7 MINUTES

4 slices rye bread

4 teaspoons reduced-fat margarine (35% vegetable oil)

1/2 cup egg substitute

1 1/2 ounces sliced, reduced-fat Swiss cheese, torn in small pieces

1   Spread one side of each bread slice with 1 teaspoon margarine and set aside.

2   Place a medium skillet over medium heat until hot. Coat with nonstick cooking spray and add the egg substitute. Cook 1 minute without stirring. Using a rubber spatula, lift up the edges to allow the uncooked portion to run under. Cook 1–2 minutes longer or until eggs are almost set and beginning to puff up slightly. Flip and cook 30 seconds.

3   Remove the skillet from the heat and spoon half of the eggs on the unbuttered sides of two of the bread slices. Arrange equal amounts of the cheese evenly over each piece and top with the remaining bread slices, buttered sides up.

4   Return the skillet to medium heat until hot. Coat the skillet with nonstick cooking spray. Add the two sandwiches and cook 3 minutes, then turn and cook 2 minutes longer or until golden brown. Using a serrated knife, cut each sandwich in half.

COOK'S TIP

To double this recipe, cook the sandwiches in two batches for best results.

EXCHANGES

2 Starch
2 Lean Meat

Calories 247
  Calories from Fat 69

Total Fat 8 g
  Saturated Fat 2.5 g

Cholesterol 8 mg

Sodium 613 mg

Total Carbohydrate 26 g
  Dietary Fiber 3 g
  Sugars 1 g

Protein 17 g

SAUSAGE–POTATO SKILLET CASSEROLE

Serves 4/Serving size: 1 cup

PREP TIME: 10 MINUTES
COOK TIME: 17 MINUTES
STAND TIME: 5 MINUTES

6 ounces reduced-fat, smoked turkey sausage, kielbasa style

2 cups chopped onion

4 cups frozen hash brown potatoes with peppers and onions

1/3 cup shredded, reduced-fat, sharp cheddar cheese

1. Cut the sausage in fourths lengthwise. Cut each piece of sausage in 1/4-inch pieces.

2. Place a large nonstick skillet over medium-high heat until hot. Coat the skillet with nonstick cooking spray, add sausage, and cook 3 minutes or until the sausage begins to brown, stirring frequently. Set the sausage aside on a separate plate.

3. Recoat the skillet with nonstick cooking spray, add the onions, and cook 5 minutes or until the onions begin to brown, stirring frequently.

4. Reduce the heat to medium, add the frozen potatoes and sausage, and cook 9 minutes or until the potatoes are lightly browned, stirring occasionally.

5. Remove the skillet from the heat, top with cheese, cover, and let stand 5 minutes to melt the cheese and develop flavors.

COOK'S TIP

The generous amount of onion adds extra moisture and texture as well as great flavor to this dish—without overpowering it!

EXCHANGES

1 1/2 Starch
2 Vegetable
1 Lean Meat

Calories 200
  Calories from Fat 38

Total Fat 4 g
  Saturated Fat 2 g

Cholesterol 26 mg

Sodium 466 mg

Total Carbohydrate 31 g
  Dietary Fiber 3 g
  Sugars 6 g

Protein 9 g

RAISIN FRENCH TOAST WITH APRICOT SPREAD

Serves 4/Serving size: 2 pieces toast plus 2 tablespoons spread

PREP TIME: 8 MINUTES PER BATCH
COOK TIME: 6 MINUTES PER BATCH

8 slices cinnamon raisin bread

3 tablespoons reduced-fat margarine (35% vegetable oil)

1/4 cup apricot or any flavor all-fruit spread

1 cup egg substitute (divided use)

1. Arrange 4 bread slices on the bottom of a 13 × 9-inch baking pan. Pour 1/2 cup egg substitute evenly over all and turn several times to coat. Let stand 2 minutes to absorb egg slightly.

2. Meanwhile, using a fork, stir the margarine and fruit spread together in a small bowl until well blended.

3. Place a large nonstick skillet over medium heat until hot. Liberally coat the skillet with nonstick cooking spray, add 4 bread slices (leaving any remaining egg mixture in the baking pan), and cook 3 minutes.

4. Turn and cook 3 minutes longer or until the bread is golden brown. For darker toast, turn the slices again and cook 1 minute more. Set aside on a serving platter and cover to keep warm.

5. While the first batch is cooking, place the remaining bread slices in the baking pan and pour the remaining egg substitute evenly over all. Turn several times to coat. Cook as directed.

6. Serve each piece of toast topped with 1 tablespoon of the margarine mixture.

COOK'S TIP

Be sure to use a fork when mixing the margarine and fruit spread together...this helps the fruit spread break down and blend evenly. The fork acts like a small whisk!

EXCHANGES
2 Starch
1/2 Fruit
1 Fat

Calories 246
  Calories from Fat 54

Total Fat 6 g
  Saturated Fat 1 g

Cholesterol 0 mg

Sodium 387 mg

Total Carbohydrate 38 g
  Dietary Fiber 2 g
  Sugars 16 g

Protein 10 g

DOUBLE-DUTY BANANA PANCAKES

Serves 4/Serving size: 2 pancakes

PREP TIME: 7 MINUTES
COOK TIME: 6 MINUTES

2 ripe medium bananas, thinly sliced

1 cup regular pancake mix

3/4 cup plus 2 tablespoons fat-free milk

4 tablespoons light pancake syrup

1 Mash one half of the banana slices and place in a medium bowl with the pancake mix and the milk. Stir until just blended.

2 Place a large nonstick skillet over medium heat until hot. (To test, sprinkle with a few drops of water. If the water drops "dance" or jump in the pan, it's hot enough.) Coat the skillet with nonstick cooking spray, add two scant 1/4 cup measures of batter, and cook the pancakes until puffed and dry around the edges, about 1 minute.

3 Flip the pancakes and cook until golden on the bottom. Place on a plate and cover to keep warm.

4 Recoat the skillet with nonstick cooking spray, add three scant 1/4 cup measures of batter, and cook as directed. Repeat with the remaining batter.

5 Place 2 pancakes on each of 4 dinner plates, top with equal amounts of banana slices, and drizzle evenly with the syrup. If you like, place the dinner plates in a warm oven and add the pancakes as they are cooked.

COOK'S TIP

The bananas in these pancakes add great flavor and fiber.

EXCHANGES
3 Carbohydrate

Calories 212
  Calories from Fat 6
Total Fat 1 g
  Saturated Fat 0 g
Cholesterol 1 mg
Sodium 627 mg
Total Carbohydrate 48 g
  Dietary Fiber 3 g
  Sugars 22 g
Protein 5 g

PEACH–CRANBERRY QUICK BREAD

Serves 12/Serving size: 1 slice

PREP TIME: 8 MINUTES
COOK TIME: 45 MINUTES
COOL TIME: 20 MINUTES

15.6-ounce box cranberry quick bread and muffin mix
1 cup water
1/2 cup egg substitute or 4 large egg whites
2 tablespoons canola oil
2 cups chopped frozen and thawed unsweetened peaches

1 Preheat the oven to 375 degrees.

2 Coat a nonstick 9 × 5-inch loaf pan with nonstick cooking spray.

3 Beat the bread mix, water, egg substitute, and oil in a medium bowl for 50 strokes or until well blended. Stir in the peaches and spoon into the loaf pan. Bake 45 minutes or until a wooden toothpick comes out clean.

4 Place the loaf pan on a wire rack for 20 minutes before removing the bread from the pan. Cool completely for peak flavor and texture.

COOK'S TIP

The peaches make this quick bread especially flavorful and moist. It freezes well, too!

EXCHANGES

2 Carbohydrate
1/2 Fat

Calories 175
  Calories from Fat 37
Total Fat 4 g
  Saturated Fat 1 g
Cholesterol 0 mg
Sodium 152 mg
Total Carbohydrate 33 g
  Dietary Fiber 1 g
  Sugars 17 g
Protein 4 g

JAM-KISSED PECAN MUFFINS

Serves 9/Serving size: 1 muffin

PREP TIME: 8 MINUTES
COOK TIME: 15 MINUTES
STAND TIME: 15 MINUTES

7-ounce box low-fat blueberry muffin mix

1/2 cup water

1/2 teaspoon ground cinnamon

1 1/2 tablespoons apricot or raspberry all-fruit spread

1 1/2 ounces pecan chips (about 1/3 cup)

1. Preheat the oven to 375 degrees.

2. Combine the muffin mix, water, and cinnamon in a medium bowl and stir until just blended. Do not overmix.

3. Place 9 foil cup liners in muffin cups and spray the liners with nonstick cooking spray. Using a measuring spoon, spoon 1 tablespoon of batter into each liner. Top each with 1/2 teaspoon jam. Top evenly with the remaining batter and sprinkle evenly with the pecans.

4. Bake 15 minutes or until a wooden toothpick comes out clean. Cool muffins in the pan on a wire rack for 15 minutes.

5. Remove the muffins from the pan and place on a wire rack to cool completely. Store in an airtight container.

COOK'S TIP

To serve warm muffins, microwave each on HIGH for 10 seconds.

EXCHANGES

1 Carbohydrate
1/2 Fat

Calories 103
　Calories from Fat 32

Total Fat 4 g
　Saturated Fat 0 g

Cholesterol 0 mg

Sodium 109 mg

Total Carbohydrate 17 g
　Dietary Fiber 2 g
　Sugars 9 g

Protein 2 g

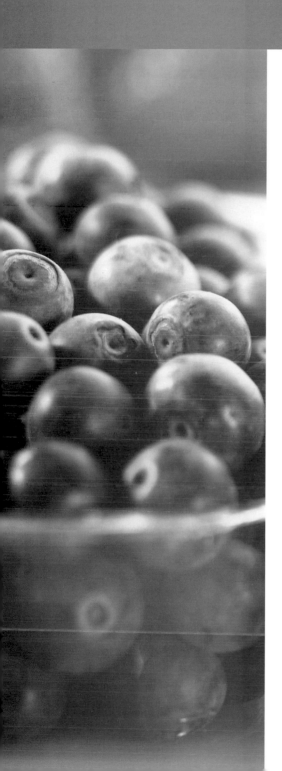

SNACKS

LIME'D BLUEBERRIES

Serves 4/Serving size: 1/2 cup

PREP TIME: 5 MINUTES

2 cups frozen unsweetened blueberries, partially thawed

1/4 cup frozen grape juice concentrate

1 1/2 tablespoons lime juice

1 Place all ingredients in a medium bowl and toss gently.

2 Serve immediately for peak flavor and texture.

COOK'S TIP

To thaw the blueberries quickly, place them in a colander and run under cold water for 20 seconds. Shake off excess liquid.

EXCHANGES

1/2 Fruit

Calories 83
  Calories from Fat 0

Total Fat 0 g
  Saturated Fat 0 g

Cholesterol 0 mg

Sodium 7 mg

Total Carbohydrate 20 g
  Dietary Fiber 2 g
  Sugars 17 g

Protein 0 g

COOK'S TIP

Whenever a recipe calls for citrus zest, such as lemon, lime, or orange, wrap the unused fruit in plastic wrap and refrigerate for a later use. You're sure to need fresh citrus juice for the next recipe!

EXCHANGES

1 Lean Meat

Calories 47
  Calories from Fat 14

Total Fat 2 g
  Saturated Fat 0 g

Cholesterol 61 mg

Sodium 141 mg

Total Carbohydrate 1 g
  Dietary Fiber 0 g
  Sugars 1 g

Protein 7 g

ZESTY LEMONY SHRIMP

Serves 8/Serving size: 1/4 cup

PREP TIME: 5 MINUTES
COOK TIME: 7–10 MINUTES

12 ounces peeled raw medium shrimp, fresh or frozen and thawed

2 tablespoons Worcestershire sauce

1 teaspoon lemon zest

3 tablespoons lemon juice

2 tablespoons reduced-fat margarine (35% vegetable oil)

1 tablespoon finely chopped fresh parsley (optional)

1 Place a large nonstick skillet over medium heat until hot. Add the shrimp, Worcestershire sauce, lemon zest, and lemon juice to the skillet. Cook 5 minutes or until shrimp is opaque in center, stirring frequently.

2 Using a slotted spoon, remove the shrimp and set aside in serving bowl. Increase the heat to medium high, add the margarine, bring to a boil, and continue to boil 2 minutes or until the liquid measures 1/4 cup, stirring constantly.

3 Pour the sauce over the shrimp and sprinkle with parsley, if desired. Serve with wooden toothpicks.

CREAMY APRICOT FRUIT DIP

Serves 4/Serving size: 2 tablespoons

PREP TIME: 5 MINUTES

1/3 cup fat-free vanilla-flavored yogurt

1/4 cup fat-free whipped topping

2 tablespoons apricot all-fruit spread

2 cups whole strawberries or 2 medium apples, halved, cored, and sliced

1 In a small bowl, whisk the yogurt, whipped topping, and fruit spread until well blended.

2 Serve with fruit.

COOK'S TIP

Squeeze a small amount of orange juice over sliced apples to prevent browning.

EXCHANGES
1 Fruit

Calories 56
  Calories from Fat 0

Total Fat 0 g
  Saturated Fat 0 g

Cholesterol 0 mg

Sodium 16 mg

Total Carbohydrate 13 g
  Dietary Fiber 2 g
  Sugars 9 g

Protein 1 g

BLEU CHEESE'D PEARS

Serves 4/Serving size: 5 pear slices with about 3/4 teaspoon cheese

PREP TIME: 5 MINUTES

2 ounces fat-free cream cheese

1/4 cup crumbled bleu cheese

2 medium firm pears, halved, cored, and sliced into 20 slices

1 In a small bowl, microwave the cheeses on HIGH for 10 seconds to soften. Use a rubber spatula to blend well.

2 Top each pear slice with 3/4 teaspoon cheese.

3 To prevent the pear slices from discoloring, toss them with a tablespoon of orange, pineapple, or lemon juice. Shake off the excess liquid before topping them with cheese.

COOK'S TIP

To make pretty hors d'oeuvres, use a small pastry bag to top each pear with cheese. Be sure to toss the pear slices with juice first to prevent discoloration.

EXCHANGES

1/2 Fruit
1/2 Fat

Calories 88
　Calories from Fat 19

Total Fat 2 g
　Saturated Fat 1 g

Cholesterol 7 mg

Sodium 200 mg

Total Carbohydrate 14 g
　Dietary Fiber 3 g
　Sugars 9 g

Protein 4 g

BASIL SPREAD AND WATER CRACKERS

Serves 4/Serving size: 1 tablespoon spread plus 3 crackers

PREP TIME: 5 MINUTES

2 ounces reduced-fat garlic and herb cream cheese

1/4 cup finely chopped fresh basil

12 fat-free water crackers

1 Stir the cream cheese and basil together in a small bowl until well blended.

2 Place 1 teaspoon spread on each cracker.

COOK'S TIP

You can stir in a small amount of milk to this cream cheese and make a delicious dip for fresh vegetables.

EXCHANGES

1/2 Starch
1/2 Fat

Calories 63
  Calories from Fat 19
Total Fat 2 g
  Saturated Fat 1 g
Cholesterol 3 mg
Sodium 125 mg
Total Carbohydrate 8 g
  Dietary Fiber 0 g
  Sugars 0 g
Protein 3 g

BABY CARROTS AND SPICY CREAM DIP

Serves 4/Serving size: 2 tablespoons dip plus 12 baby carrots

PREP TIME: 5 MINUTES
STAND TIME: 10 MINUTES

1/3 cup fat-free sour cream

3 tablespoons reduced-fat tub-style cream cheese

3/4 teaspoon hot pepper sauce

1/4 teaspoon salt

48 baby carrots

1 Stir the sour cream, cream cheese, pepper sauce, and salt together until well blended.

2 Let stand at least 10 minutes to develop flavors and mellow slightly. Serve with carrots.

COOK'S TIP

You can cover this dip with plastic wrap and refrigerate it up to 1 week.

EXCHANGES

2 Vegetable
1/2 Fat

Calories 73
  Calories from Fat 17
Total Fat 2 g
  Saturated Fat 1 g
Cholesterol 8 mg
Sodium 276 mg
Total Carbohydrate 10 g
  Dietary Fiber 3 g
  Sugars 5 g
Protein 3 g

CROSTINI WITH KALAMATA TOMATOES

Serves 4/Serving size: 3 slices crostini

PREP TIME: 10 MINUTES
COOK TIME: 10 MINUTES
STAND TIME: 10 MINUTES

4 ounces baguette bread, cut in 12 slices (about 1/4 inch thick)

1 small tomato, finely chopped

9 small kalamata olives, pitted and finely chopped

2 tablespoons chopped fresh basil

1 Preheat the oven to 350 degrees.

2 Arrange the bread slices on a baking sheet and bake 10 minutes or until just golden on the edges. Remove from the heat and cool completely.

3 Meanwhile, stir the remaining ingredients together in a small bowl. Spread 1 tablespoon of the mixture on each bread slice.

COOK'S TIP

For a thicker topping, drain the tomato mixture before spreading it on the bread.

EXCHANGES

1 Starch

Calories 90
  Calories from Fat 15

Total Fat 2 g
  Saturated Fat 0 g

Cholesterol 0 mg

Sodium 236 mg

Total Carbohydrate 16 g
  Dietary Fiber 1 g
  Sugars 1 g

Protein 3 g

COOK'S TIP

This appetizer is delicious served hot or at room temperature.

EXCHANGES

1 Vegetable

Calories 29
  Calories from Fat 11

Total Fat 1 g
  Saturated Fat 0 g

Cholesterol 0 mg

Sodium 240 mg

Total Carbohydrate 4 g
  Dietary Fiber 1 g
  Sugars 1 g

Protein 2 g

ASIAN MARINATED MUSHROOMS

Serves 4/Serving size: 4 mushrooms

PREP TIME: 5 MINUTES
MARINATE TIME: 30 MINUTES
COOK TIME: 8 MINUTES

8 ounces whole medium mushrooms, stemmed and wiped clean with damp paper towel

2 tablespoons lite soy sauce

2 tablespoons lime juice

1 teaspoon extra virgin olive oil

2 tablespoons chopped fresh parsley (optional)

1 Place the mushrooms, soy sauce, lime juice, and oil in a large plastic zippered bag. Seal the bag and shake to coat completely. Let stand 30 minutes. Meanwhile, preheat the broiler.

2 Place mushroom mixture (with marinade) in an 8-inch pie pan or baking pan and broil 4 inches away from heat source for 8 minutes or until the mushrooms begin to brown, stirring frequently.

3 Serve with wooden toothpicks and marinade.

TOMATO–CILANTRO SALSA

Serves 4/Serving size: 1/4 cup salsa plus 3/4 ounce chips

PREP TIME: 10 MINUTES

3 medium tomatoes, seeded and finely chopped

1/4 cup chopped cilantro (optional)

2 medium jalapeño peppers, stems removed, halved, seeded, and minced

3–4 tablespoons lime juice

1/4 teaspoon salt

3 ounces baked low-fat tortilla chips

1 Combine all ingredients except chips in a small bowl; serve with chips.

2 For peak flavor, serve this within 1 hour of preparing it.

COOK'S TIP

It's important to seed the tomato before chopping it—otherwise the salsa is too watery. For a milder salsa, use 1 tablespoon minced green bell pepper and 2–3 drops hot pepper sauce. Be sure to remove the seeds and membrane from the jalapeño pepper, or your salsa will be extra hot!

EXCHANGES
1 Starch
1 Vegetable

Calories 107
  Calories from Fat 8

Total Fat 1 g
  Saturated Fat 0 g

Cholesterol 0 mg

Sodium 302 mg

Total Carbohydrate 24 g
  Dietary Fiber 3 g
  Sugars 3 g

Protein 3 g

COOK'S TIP

This recipe is also delicious with honey instead of brown sugar. You can cover and refrigerate this dip for up to 5 days.

EXCHANGES

1 Fruit
1/2 Carbohydrate
1/2 Fat

Calories 120
  Calories from Fat 27

Total Fat 3 g
  Saturated Fat 1 g

Cholesterol 0 mg

Sodium 51 mg

Total Carbohydrate 22 g
  Dietary Fiber 2 g
  Sugars 12 g

Protein 3 g

SWEET PEANUT BUTTERY DIP

Serves 4/Serving size: 1/2 banana plus 2 tablespoons dip

PREP TIME: 5 MINUTES

1/3 cup fat-free vanilla-flavored yogurt

2 tablespoons reduced-fat peanut butter

2 teaspoons packed dark brown sugar

2 medium bananas, sliced

1 Using a fork or whisk, stir the yogurt, peanut butter, and brown sugar together in a small bowl until completely blended.

2 Serve with banana slices and wooden toothpicks, if desired.

DILLED CHEX TOSS

Serves 12/Serving size: 1/2 cup

PREP TIME: 5 MINUTES
COOK TIME: 30 MINUTES

6 cups multi-grain or Wheat Chex cereal

.4-ounce packet Ranch salad dressing mix

1 tablespoon dried dill

2 tablespoons extra virgin olive oil

1 Preheat the oven to 175 degrees.

2 Place the cereal, dressing mix, and dill in a large zippered plastic bag. Seal and shake gently to blend well.

3 Place the mixture on a large rimmed baking sheet or jelly roll pan, drizzle the oil evenly over all, and stir thoroughly to blend. Spread out in a single layer and bake 30 minutes or until browned lightly, stirring once.

COOK'S TIP

Store this tasty toss in an airtight container in a cool, dry area up to 2 weeks.

EXCHANGES

1 1/2 Starch

Calories 109
  Calories from Fat 26

Total Fat 3 g
  Saturated Fat 0 g

Cholesterol 0 mg

Sodium 348 mg

Total Carbohydrate 22 g
  Dietary Fiber 3 g
  Sugars 7 g

Protein 2 g

TUNA SALAD-STUFFED EGGS

Serves 4/Serving size: 2 egg halves

PREP TIME: 5 MINUTES
COOK TIME: 10 MINUTES
STAND TIME: 1 MINUTE

4 large eggs

3-ounce packet tuna (or 6-ounce can of tuna packed in water, rinsed and well drained)

2 tablespoons reduced-fat mayonnaise

1 1/2–2 tablespoons sweet pickle relish

1 Place eggs in a medium saucepan and cover with cold water. Bring to a boil over high heat, then reduce the heat and simmer 10 minutes.

2 Meanwhile, stir the tuna, mayonnaise, and relish together in a small bowl.

3 When the eggs are cooked, remove them from the water and let stand one minute before peeling under cold running water. Cut eggs in half, lengthwise, and discard 2 egg yolk halves.

4 Place the other 2 egg yolk halves in the tuna mixture and stir with a rubber spatula until well blended. Spoon equal amounts of the tuna mixture in each of the egg halves.

5 Serve immediately, or cover with plastic wrap and refrigerate up to 24 hours.

COOK'S TIP

These easy appetizers are also delicious with salmon instead of tuna. Simply use an equal amount of the salmon found in packets next to the tuna in the supermarket.

EXCHANGES

1 Lean Meat
1/2 Fat

Calories 84
  Calories from Fat 34

Total Fat 4 g
  Saturated Fat 1 g

Cholesterol 65 mg

Sodium 368 mg

Total Carbohydrate 3 g
  Dietary Fiber 0 g
  Sugars 3 g

Protein 10 g

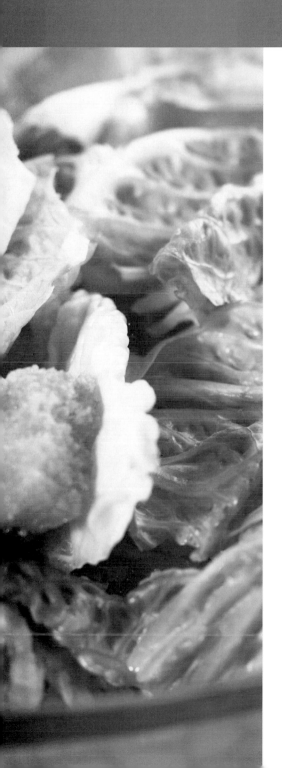

SALADS

LEMONY ASPARAGUS SPEAR SALAD

Serves 4/Serving size: 5 spears

PREP TIME: 6 MINUTES
COOK TIME: 1 MINUTE

1 pound asparagus spears, trimmed

1 tablespoon basil pesto sauce

2 teaspoons lemon juice

1/4 teaspoon salt

1 Cover asparagus with water in a large skillet and bring to a boil, then cover tightly and cook 1 minute or until tender-crisp.

2 Immediately drain the asparagus in a colander and run under cold water to cool. Place the asparagus on paper towels to drain, then place on a serving platter.

3 Top the asparagus with the pesto and roll the spears back and forth to coat completely. Drizzle with lemon juice and sprinkle with salt. Flavors are at their peak if you serve this within 30 minutes.

COOK'S TIP

You can cook the asparagus ahead of time and refrigerate it, but wait until serving time to add the remaining ingredients.

EXCHANGES

1 Vegetable
1/2 Fat

Calories 40
  Calories from Fat 19
Total Fat 2 g
  Saturated Fat 1 g
Cholesterol 1 mg
Sodium 180 mg
Total Carbohydrate 4 g
  Dietary Fiber 1 g
  Sugars 1 g
Protein 3 g

ARTICHOKE–TOMATO TOSS

Serves 4/Serving size: 1/2 cup

PREP TIME: 4 MINUTES

1/2 of a 14-ounce can quartered artichoke hearts, drained

1 cup grape tomatoes, halved

2 tablespoons fat-free Caesar or Italian dressing

2 ounces crumbled, reduced-fat, sun-dried tomato and basil feta cheese

2 tablespoons chopped fresh parsley (optional)

1 In a medium bowl, toss the artichoke hearts, tomatoes, and dressing gently, yet thoroughly. Add the feta and toss gently again.

2 Serve immediately or cover with plastic wrap and refrigerate up to 3 days.

COOK'S TIP

Toss very lightly after adding the feta for peak color and texture.

EXCHANGES

1 Vegetable
1/2 Fat

Calories 54
  Calories from Fat 19

Total Fat 2 g
  Saturated Fat 1 g

Cholesterol 4 mg

Sodium 353 mg

Total Carbohydrate 5 g
  Dietary Fiber 1 g
  Sugars 2 g

Protein 4 g

CREAMY DILL CUCUMBERS

Serves 4/Serving size: 1/2 cup

PREP TIME: 6 MINUTES

1/4 cup plain fat-free yogurt

1 tablespoon reduced-fat mayonnaise

1/2 teaspoon dried dill

1/4 teaspoon salt

2 cups peeled diced cucumber

1 Stir the yogurt, mayonnaise, dill, and salt together in a small bowl until completely blended.

2 Place the cucumbers in a medium bowl, add the yogurt mixture, and toss gently to coat completely.

3 Serve within 30 minutes for peak flavors and texture.

COOK'S TIP

For variety, try using fat-free sour cream instead of the yogurt.

EXCHANGES

1 Vegetable

Calories 30
  Calories from Fat 12

Total Fat 1 g
  Saturated Fat 0 g

Cholesterol 1 mg

Sodium 190 mg

Total Carbohydrate 3 g
  Dietary Fiber 1 g
  Sugars 2 g

Protein 1 g

BACON–ONION POTATO SALAD

Serves 4/Serving size: 1/2 cup

PREP TIME: 10 MINUTES
COOK TIME: 4 MINUTES
CHILL TIME: 2 HOURS (OPTIONAL)

12 ounces unpeeled red potatoes, diced (about 3 cups)

3 tablespoons reduced-fat Ranch salad dressing

1/2 cup finely chopped green onion

3 tablespoons real bacon bits (not imitation)

1/8 teaspoon salt

1. Bring water to boil in a medium saucepan over high heat. Add the potatoes and return to a boil. Reduce the heat, cover tightly, and cook 4 minutes or until just tender when pierced with a fork.

2. Drain the potatoes in a colander and run under cold water until cool, about 30 seconds. Drain well and place in a medium bowl with the remaining ingredients except the salt. Toss gently to blend well.

3. Serve immediately or cover with plastic wrap and refrigerate 2 hours for a more blended flavor. To serve, add the salt and toss.

COOK'S TIP

For peak flavor and texture, serve this salad the same day you make it.

EXCHANGES

1 1/2 Starch
1/2 Fat

Calories 123
  Calories from Fat 25
Total Fat 3 g
  Saturated Fat 1 g
Cholesterol 7 mg
Sodium 400 mg
Total Carbohydrate 19 g
  Dietary Fiber 2 g
  Sugars 2 g
Protein 4 g

BALSAMIC BEAN SALSA SALAD

Serves 4/Serving size: 1/2 cup

PREP TIME: 6 MINUTES
STAND TIME: 15 MINUTES

15-ounce can black beans, rinsed and drained

1/2 cup chopped red bell pepper

1/4 cup finely chopped red onion

2 tablespoons balsamic vinegar

1 Toss all ingredients in a medium bowl.

2 Let stand 15 minutes to develop flavors.

COOK'S TIP

You can cover this salad with plastic wrap and refrigerate up to 8 hours.

EXCHANGES

1 Starch

Calories 93
  Calories from Fat 0

Total Fat 0 g
  Saturated Fat 0 g

Cholesterol 0 mg

Sodium 77 mg

Total Carbohydrate 18 g
  Dietary Fiber 6 g
  Sugars 3 g

Protein 6 g

TANGY SWEET CARROT–PEPPER SALAD

Serves 4/Serving size: 1/2 cup

PREP TIME: 12 MINUTES
COOK TIME: 1 MINUTE
STAND TIME: 30 MINUTES (OPTIONAL)

1 1/2 cups peeled sliced carrots (about 1/8 inch thick)
2 tablespoons water
3/4 cup thinly sliced green bell pepper
1/3 cup thinly sliced onion
1/4 cup reduced-fat Catalina dressing

1 Place carrots and water in a shallow, microwave-safe dish, such as a glass pie plate. Cover with plastic wrap and microwave on HIGH for 1 minute or until carrots are just tender-crisp. Be careful not to overcook them—the carrots should retain some crispness.

2 Immediately place the carrots in a colander and run under cold water about 30 seconds to cool. Shake to drain and place the carrots on paper towels to dry further. Dry the dish.

3 When the carrots are completely cool, return them to the dish, add the remaining ingredients, and toss gently to coat.

4 Serve immediately, or chill 30 minutes for a more blended flavor. Flavors are at their peak if you serve this salad within 30 minutes of adding dressing.

COOK'S TIP

To make this salad ahead of time, combine the prepared carrots with the peppers and onions up to 24 hours in advance. Toss with the dressing 30 minutes before serving.

EXCHANGES

1/2 Carbohydrate
1 Vegetable

Calories 60
  Calories from Fat 6

Total Fat 1 g
  Saturated Fat 0 g

Cholesterol 0 mg

Sodium 251 mg

Total Carbohydrate 13 g
  Dietary Fiber 2 g
  Sugars 8 g

Protein 1 g

CRISPY CRUNCH COLESLAW

Serves 4/Serving size: 1/2 cup

PREP TIME: 7 MINUTES
CHILL TIME: 3 HOURS

3 cups shredded cabbage mix with carrots and red cabbage

1 medium green bell pepper, finely chopped

2–3 tablespoons apple cider vinegar

2 tablespoons sugar

1/8 teaspoon salt

1 Place all ingredients in a large zippered plastic bag, seal tightly, and shake to blend thoroughly.

2 Refrigerate 3 hours before serving to blend flavors. This salad tastes best served the same day you make it.

COOK'S TIP

For more heat, use a poblano chili pepper in place of the green bell pepper.

EXCHANGES

1/2 Carbohydrate
1 Vegetable

Calories 46
  Calories from Fat 0

Total Fat 0 g
  Saturated Fat 0 g

Cholesterol 0 mg

Sodium 90 mg

Total Carbohydrate 11 g
  Dietary Fiber 2 g
  Sugars 9 g

Protein 1 g

THOUSAND ISLE WEDGES

Serves 4/Serving size: 1 wedge plus 2 tablespoons dressing

PREP TIME: 5 MINUTES

3 tablespoons ketchup

1 tablespoon reduced-fat mayonnaise

1/4 tcaspoon salt (optional)

1/3 cup fat-free buttermilk

1/2 small head iceberg lettuce, cut in 4 wedges

Coarsely ground black pepper (optional)

1 Stir the ketchup, mayonnaise, and salt together in a small bowl until smooth. Add the buttermilk and blend thoroughly.

2 Place a lettuce wedge on each salad plate, spoon 2 tablespoons dressing on top of each wedge, and sprinkle evenly with black pepper, if desired.

COOK'S TIP

Be sure to combine the ingredients as direcled before adding the buttermilk—otherwise it's difficult to remove the lumps! You won't believe how much better this Thousand Island dressing tastes than the store-bought versions.

EXCHANGES

1 Vegetable
1/2 Fat

Calories 42
  Calories from Fat 14

Total Fat 2 g
  Saturated Fat 0 g

Cholesterol 2 mg

Sodium 192 mg

Total Carbohydrate 6 g
  Dietary Fiber 1 g
  Sugars 3 g

Protein 2 g

MILD MUSTARD ROMAINE SALAD

Serves 4/Serving size: 2 cups salad plus 2 tablespoons dressing

PREP TIME: 5 MINUTES

1/2 cup fat-free sour cream

2 tablespoons water

2 teaspoons prepared mustard

2 teaspoons reduced-fat mayonnaise

1/2 teaspoon salt

8 cups packed torn Romaine lettuce

Coarsely ground black pepper to taste (optional)

1 Stir the sour cream, water, mustard, mayonnaise, and salt together in a small bowl until well blended.

2 Place the lettuce in a large bowl, add the dressing, and toss gently to coat. Sprinkle with black pepper, if desired.

COOK'S TIP

For peak flavor, be sure to toss this salad thoroughly to evenly coat the lettuce.

EXCHANGES

1 Vegetable
1/2 Fat

Calories 43
  Calories from Fat 9

Total Fat 1 g
  Saturated Fat 0 g

Cholesterol 4 mg

Sodium 359 mg

Total Carbohydrate 3 g
  Dietary Fiber 1 g
  Sugars 2 g

Protein 3 g

CUMIN'D PICANTE SALAD

Serves 4/Serving size: 2 cups

PREP TIME: 3 MINUTES

3/4 cup mild or medium picante sauce

2 tablespoons water

1/4 teaspoon ground cumin

8 cups shredded lettuce

20 baked bite-sized tortilla chips, coarsely crumbled
(1 ounce)

1 Stir the picante sauce, water, and cumin together in a small bowl.

2 Place 2 cups of lettuce on each of 4 salad plates, spoon 3 tablespoons picante mixture over each salad, and top with chips.

COOK'S TIP

For variation, add 1 cup diced cucumber or matchstick carrots to the shredded lettuce.

EXCHANGES

1/2 Starch
1 Vegetable

Calories 53
  Calories from Fat 0
Total Fat 0 g
  Saturated Fat 0 g
Cholesterol 0 mg
Sodium 446 mg
Total Carbohydrate 11 g
  Dietary Fiber 2 g
  Sugars 1 g
Protein 2 g

PEAR AND BLEU CHEESE GREENS

Serves 4/Serving size: 2 cups

PREP TIME: 4 MINUTES

6 cups spring greens

2 cups firm pear slices or green apple slices

1/2 cup fat-free raspberry vinaigrette

3–4 tablespoons crumbled reduced-fat bleu cheese

1   Place 1 1/2 cups of the greens on each of 4 salad plates. Arrange 1/2 cup apple slices on each serving.

2   Top with 2 tablespoons dressing and 1 tablespoon of the cheese. Serve immediately.

COOK'S TIP

This recipe is also delicious made with fresh berries and goat cheese (cut in small pieces).

EXCHANGES

1 Carbohydrate
1/2 Fat

Calories 96
  Calories from Fat 18

Total Fat 2 g
  Saturated Fat 1 g

Cholesterol 5 mg

Sodium 273 mg

Total Carbohydrate 19 g
  Dietary Fiber 2 g
  Sugars 14 g

Protein 2 g

COOK'S TIP

No leftover chicken? Cook 1 pound chicken breast meat in the micro-wave. Place the chicken on a microwave-safe plate, cover with plastic wrap, and cook on HIGH 2 minutes. Turn and cook 1–2 minutes longer or until the chicken is barely pink in the center. Remove and let stand 15 minutes to cool completely, then cut into bite-sized pieces.

EXCHANGES

1/2 Carbohydrate
3 Lean Meat

Calories 168
   Calories from Fat 28
Total Fat 3 g
   Saturated Fat 1 g
Cholesterol 74 mg
Sodium 274 mg
Total Carbohydrate 5 g
   Dietary Fiber 0 g
   Sugars 2 g
Protein 28 g

CAESAR'D CHICKEN SALAD

Serves 4/Serving size: 1/2 cup

PREP TIME: 5 MINUTES
CHILL TIME: 2 HOURS

1/4 cup fat-free mayonnaise

3 tablespoons fat-free Caesar salad dressing

2 1/2 cups cooked diced chicken breast

1/2 cup finely chopped green onion (green and white parts)

Black pepper to taste

1 Stir the mayonnaise and salad dressing together in a medium bowl. Add the chicken, onions, and black pepper and stir until well coated.

2 Cover with plastic wrap and refrigerate at least 2 hours to allow flavors to blend. You may refrigerate this salad up to 24 hours before serving.

FETA'D TUNA WITH GREENS

Serves 4/Serving size: 1 1/2 cups

PREP TIME: 6 MINUTES

6 cups torn Boston Bibb lettuce, red leaf lettuce, or spring greens

3 tablespoons fat-free Caesar salad dressing

2 ounces crumbled, reduced-fat, sun-dried tomato and basil feta cheese

7.06 ounce packet tuna, broken in large chunks

1 Place the lettuce and salad dressing in a large bowl and toss gently, yet thoroughly, to coat completely.

2 Place 1 1/2 cups of lettuce on each of 4 salad plates. Sprinkle each salad with 1 tablespoon feta and lightly flake equal amounts of tuna in the center of each serving.

COOK'S TIP

Don't underestimate the importance of tossing the lettuce and dressing together first—it balances the recipe's flavors. The tuna packet works better in this recipe than canned tuna would—the packet tuna flakes perfectly over the well-dressed salad.

EXCHANGES
2 Lean Meat

Calories 97
  Calories from Fat 21
Total Fat 2 g
  Saturated Fat 1 g
Cholesterol 27 mg
Sodium 556 mg
Total Carbohydrate 3 g
  Dietary Fiber 1 g
  Sugars 1 g
Protein 16 g

SEASIDE SHRIMP SALAD

Serves 4/Serving size: rounded 1/2 cup

PREP TIME: 6 MINUTES
COOK TIME: 5 MINUTES
STAND TIME: 10 MINUTES
CHILL TIME: 2 HOURS

1 1/2 pounds peeled raw fresh or frozen and thawed shrimp

2 tablespoons reduced-fat mayonnaise

1 1/2 teaspoons seafood seasoning

6 tablespoons lemon juice

1 Bring water to boil in a large saucepan over high heat. Add the shrimp and return to a boil. Reduce the heat and simmer, uncovered, 2–3 minutes or until the shrimp is opaque in the center.

2 Drain the shrimp in a colander, rinse with cold water for 30 seconds, and pat dry with paper towels. Let stand 10 minutes to cool completely.

3 Place shrimp in a medium bowl with the mayonnaise, seafood seasoning, and lemon juice. Stir gently to coat. Cover with plastic wrap and refrigerate 2 hours. Serve as is or over tomato slices or lettuce leaves.

COOK'S TIP

For added lemon flavor, add 1/2 teaspoon lemon zest along with the lemon juice.

EXCHANGES

3 Lean Meat

Calories 150
  Calories from Fat 34

Total Fat 4 g
  Saturated Fat 1 g

Cholesterol 244 mg

Sodium 591 mg

Total Carbohydrate 2 g
  Dietary Fiber 0 g
  Sugars 1 g

Protein 26 g

GINGER'D AMBROSIA

Serves 4/Serving size: 1/4 recipe

PREP TIME: 12 MINUTES
STAND TIME: 5–10 MINUTES

3 medium navel oranges, peeled and cut into bite-sized sections (about 1 1/2 cups total)

3 tablespoons flaked, sweetened, shredded coconut

2–3 teaspoons grated gingerroot

1 teaspoon pourable sugar substitute (optional)

4 fresh or canned pineapple slices, packed in juice, drained

1 Place all ingredients except the pineapple in a medium bowl and toss gently. Let stand 5–10 minutes to develop flavors.

2 Arrange each pineapple slice on a salad plate and spoon a rounded 1/3 cup of the orange mixture on each slice.

COOK'S TIP

You can find orange sections in the refrigerated produce section of your supermarket, but the degree of sweetness may vary slightly.

EXCHANGES

1 Fruit

Calories 70
 Calories from Fat 11

Total Fat 1 g
 Saturated Fat 1 g

Cholesterol 0 mg

Sodium 9 mg

Total Carbohydrate 15 g
 Dietary Fiber 2 g
 Sugars 13 g

Protein 1 g

ZESTY CITRUS MELON

Serves 4/Serving size: 3/4 cup

PREP TIME: 5 MINUTES

1/4 cup orange juice

1/4–1/2 teaspoon lemon zest (optional)

2–3 tablespoons lemon juice

1 tablespoon honey

3 cups diced honeydew or cantaloupe melon

1 Stir the orange juice, lemon zest (if using), lemon juice, and honey together in a small bowl.

2 Place the melon on a serving plate and pour the juice mixture evenly over all. For peak flavor, serve within 1 hour.

COOK'S TIP

Try using half cantaloupe and half honeydew in this recipe.

EXCHANGES

1 Fruit

Calories 67
  Calories from Fat 0

Total Fat 0 g
  Saturated Fat 0 g

Cholesterol 0 mg

Sodium 13 mg

Total Carbohydrate 16 g
  Dietary Fiber 1 g
  Sugars 15 g

Protein 1 g

TOASTED PECAN AND APPLE SALAD

Serves 4/Serving size: 1/2 cup

PREP TIME: 8 MINUTES

2 tablespoons pecan chips

2 cups chopped unpeeled red apples

1/4 cup dried raisin-cherry blend (or 1/4 cup dried cherries or golden raisins alone)

1 teaspoon honey (or 1 teaspoon packed dark brown sugar and 1 teaspoon water)

4 lettuce leaves (optional)

1 Place a small skillet over medium-high heat until hot. Add the pecans and cook 1–2 minutes or until beginning to lightly brown, stirring constantly. Remove from the heat and set aside on paper towels to stop the cooking process and cool quickly.

2 Combine the apples and dried fruit in a medium bowl, drizzle honey over all, and toss gently.

3 Serve on a lettuce leaf (if using) or a pretty salad plate. Sprinkle each serving evenly with the pecans.

COOK'S TIP

Using pecan chips rather than pieces makes the nutty flavors "stretch" further in the salad. If chips are unavailable, place pecan pieces in a small zippered plastic bag and crush slightly by tapping the pieces with the back of a heavy spoon. This releases the nutty flavor.

EXCHANGES

1 Fruit
1/2 Fat

Calories 87
  Calories from Fat 25

Total Fat 3 g
  Saturated Fat 0 g

Cholesterol 0 mg

Sodium 2 mg

Total Carbohydrate 17 g
  Dietary Fiber 2 g
  Sugars 13 g

Protein 1 g

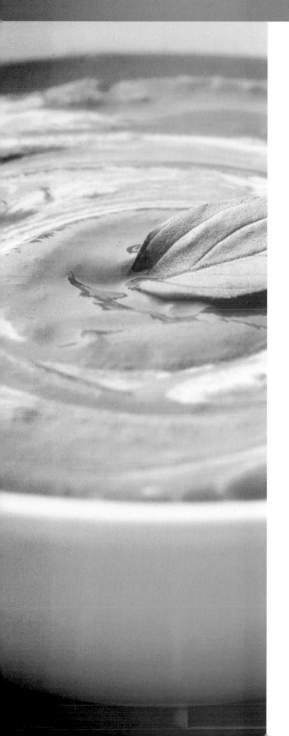

SOUPS

CHINESE STARTER SOUP

Serves 4/Serving size: 1 cup

PREP TIME: 4 MINUTES
COOK TIME: 10 MINUTES
STAND TIME: 3 MINUTES

3 cups low-fat, low-sodium chicken broth

8 ounces frozen stir-fry vegetables, such as a mix of broccoli, carrots, water chestnuts, and onion

2 teaspoons grated gingerroot

2 teaspoons lite soy sauce

1/8 teaspoon dried red pepper flakes (optional)

1 In a medium saucepan, bring the broth to boil over high heat. Add the vegetables and return to a boil.

2 Reduce the heat, cover tightly, and simmer 3–4 minutes or until vegetables are tender-crisp.

3 Remove from the heat and add the remaining ingredients. Cover and let stand 3 minutes to develop flavors, then serve.

COOK'S TIP

This soup is best served immediately, when flavors and texture are at their peak.

EXCHANGES

1 Vegetable

Calories 34
    Calories from Fat 0
Total Fat 0 g
    Saturated Fat 0 g
Cholesterol 0 mg
Sodium 487 mg
Total Carbohydrate 4 g
    Dietary Fiber 1 g
    Sugars 3 g
Protein 3 g

SMOKY TOMATO–PEPPER SOUP

Serves 4/Serving size: 1 cup

PREP TIME: 5 MINUTES
COOK TIME: 32 MINUTES

14.5-ounce can stewed tomatoes

8 ounces frozen pepper and onion stir-fry

1/2–1 medium chipotle chili pepper in adobo sauce,
mashed with a fork and then finely chopped
(1 1/2 teaspoons to 1 tablespoon total)

1 cup water

15.5-ounce can navy beans, rinsed and drained

1/4 teaspoon salt

1. In a large saucepan, combine the tomatoes, peppers, chipotle pepper, and water. Bring to a boil over high heat.

2. Reduce the heat, cover tightly, and simmer 25 minutes or until onions are tender, stirring occasionally.

3. Mash the larger pieces of tomato with a fork, then add the beans and salt and cook 5 minutes longer.

COOK'S TIP

This is a very spicy dish made with half a chipotle pepper—for a milder flavor, use less.

EXCHANGES

1 1/2 Starch
2 Vegetable

Calories 151
  Calories from Fat 7
Total Fat 1 g
  Saturated Fat 0 g
Cholesterol 0 mg
Sodium 590 mg
Total Carbohydrate 30 g
  Dietary Fiber 6 g
  Sugars 6 g
Protein 8 g

VERY VEGGIE SOUP

Serves 4/Serving size: 1 cup

PREP TIME: 2 MINUTES
COOK TIME: 15 MINUTES
STAND TIME: 5 MINUTES

4 ounces 50% reduced-fat pork breakfast sausage

2 cups coarsely chopped green cabbage
(about 3/4-inch pieces)

10-ounce package frozen mixed vegetables

14.5-ounce can stewed tomatoes with liquid

1 1/2 cups water

1 Place a large saucepan over medium-high heat until hot. Coat pan with nonstick cooking spray and add the sausage. Cook the sausage until no longer pink, stirring constantly, breaking up large pieces while cooking. Set aside on separate plate.

2 Recoat the pan with nonstick cooking spray, add the cabbage, and cook 3 minutes, stirring frequently. Add the remaining ingredients and bring to a boil. Reduce the heat, cover tightly, and simmer 10 minutes or until vegetables are tender.

3 Remove from the heat, stir in the sausage, cover, and let stand 5 minutes to develop flavors.

COOK'S TIP

This is a great recipe to double and freeze in 1-cup quantities for a quick meal. Reheat in the microwave on HIGH for 3 minutes, stir, and cook 1 minute longer or until thoroughly heated.

EXCHANGES

4 Vegetable
1 Fat

Calories 143
    Calories from Fat 55

Total Fat 6 g
    Saturated Fat 2 g

Cholesterol 19 mg

Sodium 485 mg

Total Carbohydrate 18 g
    Dietary Fiber 4 g
    Sugars 7 g

Protein 8 g

GREEN PEPPER SKILLET CHILI

Serves 4/Serving size: 1 cup

PREP TIME: 5 MINUTES
COOK TIME: 25 MINUTES
STAND TIME: 10 MINUTES

1 pound 90% lean ground beef

1 large green bell pepper, chopped (about 1 1/2 cups total)

14.5-ounce can stewed tomatoes with liquid

1.25-ounce packet chili seasoning mix

3/4 cup water

1   Place a large nonstick skillet over medium-high heat until hot. Coat the skillet with nonstick cooking spray, add the beef, and cook until no longer pink, stirring frequently. Set aside on a separate plate.

2   Recoat the skillet with nonstick cooking spray, add the peppers, and cook 5 minutes or until the edges begin to brown, stirring frequently.

3   Add the remaining ingredients to the skillet and bring to a boil. Reduce the heat, cover tightly, and simmer 15 minutes or until peppers are very tender, stirring occasionally, using the back of a spoon to crush the tomatoes while cooking.

4   Remove from the heat and let stand 10 minutes to develop flavors.

COOK'S TIP

Be sure to use the stewed variety of tomatoes in this recipe—their sweetness cuts the acidity of the tomatoes and provides additional flavor.

EXCHANGES

3 Vegetable
3 Lean Meat

Calories 244
   Calories from Fat 90

Total Fat 10 g
   Saturated Fat 4 g

Cholesterol 69 mg

Sodium 634 mg

Total Carbohydrate 14 g
   Dietary Fiber 4 g
   Sugars 4 g

Protein 24 g

SWEET CORN AND PEPPERS SOUP

Serves 5/Serving size: 1 cup

PREP TIME: 5 MINUTES
COOK TIME: 20 MINUTES
STAND TIME: 5 MINUTES

1 cup water

1 pound frozen pepper and onion stir-fry

10 ounces frozen corn kernels, thawed

1 1/4 cups fat-free milk

2 ounces reduced-fat processed cheese (such as Velveeta)
cut in small cubes

1/2 teaspoon salt

1/8 teaspoon black pepper

1   In a large saucepan, bring the water to boil over high
    heat. Add the peppers and return to a boil. Reduce the
heat, cover tightly, and simmer 15 minutes or until onions
are tender.

2   Add the corn and milk. Increase the heat to high, bring
    just to a boil, and remove from the heat.

3   Add the remaining ingredients, cover, and let stand 5
    minutes to melt the cheese and develop flavors.

COOK'S TIP

Be sure to add the
cheese after you've
removed the saucepan
from the heat; otherwise,
the cheese will curdle.

EXCHANGES
1 1/2 Carbohydrate

Calories 117
    Calories from Fat 15

Total Fat 2 g
    Saturated Fat 1 g

Cholesterol 5 mg

Sodium 438 mg

Total Carbohydrate 21 g
    Dietary Fiber 2 g
    Sugars 8 g

Protein 7 g

CREAMY POTATO SOUP WITH GREEN ONIONS

Serves 3/Serving size: 1 cup

PREP TIME: 10 MINUTES
COOK TIME: 15 MINUTES

2 cups fat-free milk

1 pound baking potatoes, peeled and diced

3 tablespoons reduced-fat margarine (35% vegetable oil)

1/2 teaspoon salt

1/4 teaspoon black pepper

3 tablespoons finely chopped green onions, green and white parts

1 Bring the milk just to a boil in a large saucepan over high heat (catch it before it comes to a full boil).

2 Add the potatoes and return just to a boil. Reduce the heat, cover tightly, and simmer 12 minutes or until the potatoes are tender.

3 Remove from the heat and add the margarine, salt, and pepper. Using a whisk or potato masher or handheld electric mixer, mash the mixture until thickened, but still lumpy.

4 Spoon into individual bowls and sprinkle each serving with 1 tablespoon onions.

COOK'S TIP

For a more colorful soup, use Yukon Gold potatoes.

EXCHANGES

1 1/2 Starch
1/2 Fat-Free Milk
1 Fat

Calories 204
  Calories from Fat 47

Total Fat 5 g
  Saturated Fat 1 g

Cholesterol 3 mg

Sodium 552 mg

Total Carbohydrate 32 g
  Dietary Fiber 2 g
  Sugars 10 g

Protein 8 g

TILAPIA STEW WITH GREEN PEPPERS

Serves 4/Serving size: 1 cup

PREP TIME: 10 MINUTES
COOK TIME: 40 MINUTES
STAND TIME: 10 MINUTES

1 medium green bell pepper, chopped

14.5-ounce can stewed tomatoes with Italian seasonings

1 cup water

1 pound tilapia filets, rinsed and cut into 1-inch pieces

3/4 teaspoon seafood seasoning

1/8 teaspoon salt

1   Place a large saucepan over medium heat until hot. Coat the pan with nonstick cooking spray, add the bell pepper, and cook 5 minutes or until beginning to lightly brown, stirring frequently.

2   Add the tomatoes and water, increase to high heat, and bring to a boil. Reduce the heat, cover tightly, and simmer 25 minutes or until the tomatoes are tender. Using the back of a spoon, break up the larger pieces of tomato.

3   Add the fish and seasonings and stir very gently. Increase the heat to high and bring just to a boil. Reduce the heat, cover tightly, and simmer 3 minutes or until the fish is opaque in the center. Remove from the heat and let stand, covered, 10 minutes to develop flavors.

COOK'S TIP

Be careful not to overstir the stew after adding the fish, or it will flake too much and change the texture and appearance of the stew.

EXCHANGES

1 Vegetable
3 Lean Meat

Calories 147
   Calories from Fat 25

Total Fat 3 g
   Saturated Fat 1 g

Cholesterol 76 mg

Sodium 460 mg

Total Carbohydrate 8 g
   Dietary Fiber 2 g
   Sugars 5 g

Protein 24 g

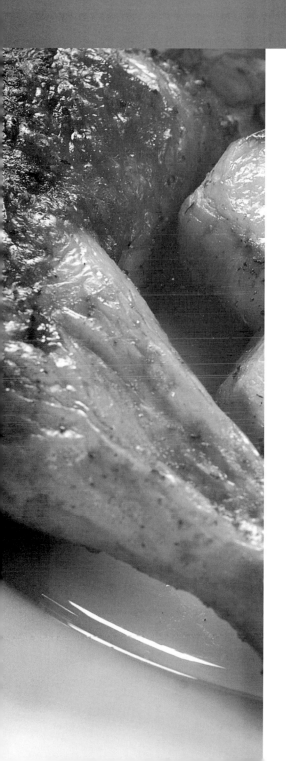

POULTRY

PEACH BARBECUED CHICKEN

Serves 4/Serving size: 2 drumsticks

PREP TIME: 15 MINUTES
COOK TIME: 18 MINUTES

8 chicken drumsticks, skin removed, rinsed and patted dry
(about 2 pounds total)

1/4 cup peach all-fruit spread

1/2 cup barbeque sauce, preferably hickory- or mesquite-flavored

2 teaspoons grated gingerroot

1 Preheat the broiler.

2 Coat a broiler rack and pan with nonstick cooking
spray. Arrange the drumsticks on the rack and broil
about 4 inches away from heat source for 8 minutes. Turn
and broil 6 minutes or until the juices run clear.

3 Meanwhile, place the fruit spread in a small glass bowl
and microwave on HIGH 20 seconds or until the fruit
spread has melted slightly. Add the barbeque sauce and
ginger and stir to blend. Place 2 tablespoons of the mixture
in a separate small bowl and set aside.

4 When the chicken is cooked, brush with half of the
sauce and broil 2 minutes. Turn the drumsticks, brush
with the remaining half of the sauce, and broil 2 more
minutes.

5 Remove the drumsticks from the broiler, turn them over,
and brush with the reserved 2 tablespoons sauce to serve.

COOK'S TIP

For easy cleanup, line
the broiler rack and pan
with foil and cut slits
in the rack foil to allow
the grease to drip down
onto the broiler pan.

EXCHANGES

1 1/2 Carbohydrate
3 Lean Meat

Calories 239
  Calories from Fat 46
Total Fat 5 g
  Saturated Fat 1 g
Cholesterol 82 mg
Sodium 438 mg
Total Carbohydrate 22 g
  Dietary Fiber 0 g
  Sugars 16 g
Protein 25 g

GREEK CHICKEN WITH LEMON

Serves 4/Serving size: 2 drumsticks

PREP TIME: 15 MINUTES
MARINATE TIME: 8 HOURS
COOK TIME: 50 MINUTES

8 chicken drumsticks, skin removed, rinsed and patted dry

2 tablespoons dried Greek seasoning
(sold in jars in the spice aisle)

2 teaspoons extra virgin olive oil

1 teaspoon lemon zest

1/2 teaspoon salt (optional)

4 tablespoons lemon juice (divided use)

1. Place the drumsticks, Greek seasoning, olive oil, lemon zest, and 2 tablespoons lemon juice in a gallon-sized zippered plastic bag. Seal the bag and toss back and forth to coat the chicken evenly. Refrigerate for 8 hours or up to 48 hours, turning occasionally.

2. Preheat the oven to 350 degrees.

3. Coat a 12 × 8-inch baking dish with nonstick cooking spray, arrange the drumsticks in a single layer, and pour the marinade evenly over all. Bake uncovered for 50–55 minutes or until the drumsticks are no longer pink in the center, turning occasionally.

4. Place the drumsticks on a serving platter. Add the salt (if using) and 2 tablespoons lemon juice to a small bowl, stir to blend well, and pour evenly over the chicken pieces.

COOK'S TIP

To skin the drumsticks easily and quickly, use one paper towel per drumstick. Grab the skin with the paper towel and pull. You'll get great traction and the chicken skin won't slip between your fingers!

EXCHANGES

3 Lean Meat

Calories 179
  Calories from Fat 67

Total Fat 7 g
  Saturated Fat 2 g

Cholesterol 82 mg

Sodium 87 mg

Total Carbohydrate 2 g
  Dietary Fiber 1 g
  Sugars 1 g

Protein 25 g

TACO CHICKEN TENDERS

Serves 4/Serving size: 3 ounces

PREP TIME: 5 MINUTES
COOK TIME: 7 MINUTES
STAND TIME: 1 MINUTE

4 teaspoons taco seasoning mix (available in packets)

1 pound chicken tenderloins, rinsed and patted dry

1/2 medium lime

2 tablespoons fat-free sour cream

1 Sprinkle the taco seasoning evenly over both sides of the chicken pieces, pressing down gently so the spices adhere.

2 Place a large nonstick skillet over medium-high heat until hot. Coat the skillet with nonstick cooking spray, add the chicken, and cook 2 minutes.

3 Turn gently to keep the seasonings on the chicken as much as possible, reduce the heat to medium, and cook 2 minutes. Turn gently and cook 2 more minutes or until the chicken is no longer pink in the center.

4 Remove from the heat, squeeze lime juice evenly over all, and serve with 1/2 tablespoon sour cream per serving.

COOK'S TIP

Store the remaining taco seasoning mix in a small zippered plastic bag in the pantry for later use.

EXCHANGES

3 Lean Meat

Calories 144
  Calories from Fat 25
Total Fat 3 g
  Saturated Fat 1 g
Cholesterol 67 mg
Sodium 281 mg
Total Carbohydrate 2 g
  Dietary Fiber 0 g
  Sugars 1 g
Protein 25 g

DIJON'D CHICKEN WITH ROSEMARY

Serves 4/Serving size: 3 ounces

PREP TIME: 5 MINUTES
COOK TIME: 13 MINUTES

1 tablespoon Dijon mustard

1 tablespoon extra virgin olive oil

1/4 teaspoon dried rosemary

4 4-ounce boneless, skinless chicken breasts, rinsed and patted dry

1. Using a fork, stir the mustard, olive oil, and rosemary together in a small bowl until well blended and set aside.

2. Place a medium nonstick skillet over medium heat until hot. Coat the skillet with nonstick cooking spray, add the chicken, and cook 5 minutes.

3. Turn the chicken, then spoon equal amounts of the mustard mixture over each piece. Reduce the heat to medium low, cover tightly, and cook 7 minutes or until the chicken is no longer pink in the center.

4. Turn the chicken several times to blend the mustard mixture with the pan drippings, place the chicken on a serving platter, and spoon the mustard mixture over all.

COOK'S TIP

For a more flavorful dish, crush the rosemary leaves before adding them to the mustard and oil.

EXCHANGES
3 Lean Meat

Calories 162
   Calories from Fat 56

Total Fat 6 g
   Saturated Fat 1 g

Cholesterol 66 mg

Sodium 147 mg

Total Carbohydrate 1 g
   Dietary Fiber 0 g
   Sugars 0 g

Protein 24 g

CHEESY CHICKEN AND RICE

Serves 4/Serving size: 1 1/2 cups

PREP TIME: 10 MINUTES
COOK TIME: 12 MINUTES

1 1/2 cups water

1 cup instant brown rice

12 ounces frozen broccoli and cauliflower florets

12 ounces boneless, skinless chicken breast, rinsed and patted dry, cut into bite-sized pieces

4 ounces reduced-fat processed cheese (such as Velveeta), cut in 1/2-inch cubes

1/4 teaspoon salt

Black pepper to taste

1 Bring the water to boil in a large saucepan, then add the rice and vegetables. Return to a boil, reduce the heat, cover tightly, and simmer 10 minutes or until the liquid is absorbed.

2 Meanwhile, place a large nonstick skillet over medium heat until hot. Coat the skillet with nonstick cooking spray and add the chicken. Cook 10 minutes or until the chicken is no longer pink in the center and is just beginning to lightly brown on the edges, stirring frequently.

3 Add the chicken, cheese, salt, and pepper to the rice mixture and stir until the cheese has melted.

COOK'S TIP

You can use reduced-fat American cheese instead of the processed cheese if you prefer.

EXCHANGES

1 1/2 Starch
1 Vegetable
3 Lean Meat

Calories 346
  Calories from Fat 59

Total Fat 7 g
  Saturated Fat 2.6 g

Cholesterol 59 mg

Sodium 654 mg

Total Carbohydrate 43 g
  Dietary Fiber 4 g
  Sugars 4 g

Protein 30 g

Serves 4/Serving size: 2 drumsticks

PREP TIME: 10 MINUTES
MARINATE TIME: 2 HOURS
COOK TIME: 25 MINUTES
STAND TIME: 3 MINUTES

1/4 cup lite soy sauce

2 tablespoons lime juice

8 chicken drumsticks, skin removed, rinsed, and patted dry

2 tablespoons dark molasses

1. Stir the soy sauce and lime juice together in a small bowl until well blended.

2. Place the drumsticks in a large zippered plastic bag. Add 3 tablespoons of the soy sauce mixture to the bag. Seal tightly and shake back and forth to coat chicken evenly. Refrigerate overnight or at least 2 hours, turning occasionally.

3. Add the molasses to the remaining soy sauce mixture, cover with plastic wrap, and refrigerate until needed.

4. Preheat the broiler. Lightly coat the broiler rack and pan with nonstick cooking spray, place the drumsticks on the rack, and discard any marinade in the bag. Broil 6 inches away from the heat source for 25 minutes, turning every 5 minutes or until the drumsticks are no longer pink in the center.

5. Place the drumsticks in a large bowl. Stir the reserved soy sauce mixture and pour it over the drumsticks. Toss the drumsticks gently to coat evenly and let them stand 3 minutes to develop flavors.

COOK'S TIP

These drumsticks are best served immediately.

EXCHANGES

1/2 Carbohydrate
3 Lean Meat

Calories 226
  Calories from Fat 56
Total Fat 6 g
  Saturated Fat 2 g
Cholesterol 102 mg
Sodium 538 mg
Total Carbohydrate 8 g
  Dietary Fiber 0 g
  Sugars 7 g
Protein 32 g

COUNTRY ROAST CHICKEN WITH LEMONY AU JUS

Serves 6/Serving size: 3 ounces

PREP TIME: 20 MINUTES
COOK TIME: 1 HOUR AND 20 MINUTES
STAND TIME: 15–20 MINUTES

3 1/2-pound roasting chicken, rinsed and patted dry, including the cavity

2 medium lemons, quartered

3/4 teaspoon poultry seasoning

3/4 teaspoon garlic powder

3/4 teaspoon salt

1/4 teaspoon black pepper

2 cups water

1 Preheat the oven to 425 degrees.

2 Coat a broiler rack and pan with nonstick cooking spray. Place the chicken on the rack. Squeeze the lemons evenly over the chicken and place the lemon rinds in the cavity of the chicken.

3 Combine the poultry seasoning, garlic powder, salt, and pepper in a small bowl. Blend well and sprinkle evenly over the chicken. Place the chicken in the oven, pour the water through the slits of the broiler pan, and cook 30 minutes.

EXCHANGES
3 Lean Meat

Calories 265
  Calories from Fat 57
Total Fat 6 g
  Saturated Fat 2 g
Cholesterol 76 mg
Sodium 174 mg
Total Carbohydrate 1 g
  Dietary Fiber 0 g
  Sugars 0 g
Protein 25 g

COOK'S TIP

If you use a zippered plastic bag to separate the grease, first pour the pan drippings into a 2-cup measuring cup, then into the bag. To remove the grease, hold the bag over a small glass bowl or saucepan, snip off a bottom corner of the bag, and allow the juice to run out, stopping when the grease is all that is left in the bag.

4 Reduce the heat to 375 degrees and cook 50–55 minutes or until a meat thermometer reaches 180 degrees. Remove the chicken from the oven and let it stand on the broiler rack for 10 minutes.

5 Place the chicken on a cutting board. Carefully pour the pan drippings into a grease separator or a plastic zippered bag. Freeze the drippings for 10 minutes to separate the grease.

6 Remove the grease from the separator or bag, pour into a glass dish, and heat in the microwave on HIGH for 30 seconds. Slice the chicken, discarding the skin, and serve with the drippings.

SEARED CHICKEN WITH SPICY CHIPOTLE CREAM SAUCE

Serves 4/Serving size: 3 ounces

PREP TIME: 8 MINUTES
COOK TIME: 14 MINUTES

4 4-ounce boneless, skinless chicken breasts, rinsed and patted dry

1/2 teaspoon salt (divided use)

1/3 cup water

6 tablespoons fat-free sour cream

2 tablespoons reduced-fat mayonnaise

1/4–1/2 medium chipotle chili pepper in adobo sauce, mashed with a fork and then finely chopped
(3/4 teaspoon to 1 1/2 teaspoons total)

1 Season the chicken with 1/4 teaspoon salt. Place a large nonstick skillet over medium-high heat until hot. Coat the skillet with nonstick cooking spray, add the chicken (smooth side down), and cook 3 minutes or until beginning to richly brown.

2 Turn the chicken and pour the water around the chicken pieces. Reduce the heat to medium, cover tightly, and cook 10 minutes or until the chicken is no longer pink in the center.

3 Meanwhile, stir the sour cream, mayonnaise, chipotle pepper, and 1/4 teaspoon salt together in a small bowl.

EXCHANGES
3 Lean Meat

Calories 169
  Calories from Fat 46
Total Fat 5 g
  Saturated Fat 1 g
Cholesterol 70 mg
Sodium 436 mg
Total Carbohydrate 2 g
  Dietary Fiber 0 g
  Sugars 1 g
Protein 26 g

COOK'S TIP

This is a very spicy dish made with half a chipotle pepper—for a milder flavor, use less.

4 Remove the skillet from the heat and place the chicken on a serving platter. Cover the chicken with foil to keep warm.

5 Reduce the heat to medium low and return the skillet to the stove. Add the sour cream mixture and stir until well blended. Cook 1 minute or until thoroughly heated, stirring constantly. Be careful not to bring the sauce to a boil, or it will separate. Spoon about 2 tablespoons of sauce over each chicken breast to serve.

WHITE WINE'D CHICKEN AND MUSHROOMS

Serves 4/Serving size: 3 ounces chicken plus 1/4 cup mushrooms

PREP TIME: 5 MINUTES
COOK TIME: 25 MINUTES

1 cup sliced mushrooms

1/4 teaspoon salt (divided use)

4 4-ounce boneless, skinless chicken breasts, rinsed and patted dry

1/8 teaspoon black pepper

1/4 teaspoon dried rosemary, crushed (optional)

1/2 cup dry white wine

2 tablespoons reduced-fat margarine (35% vegetable oil)

1 Place a large nonstick skillet over medium-high heat until hot. Coat the skillet with nonstick cooking spray and add the mushrooms and 1/8 teaspoon salt. Cook for 5 minutes or until the mushrooms begin to richly brown on the edges, stirring frequently. Set the mushrooms aside on a separate plate.

2 Sprinkle the chicken with the remaining 1/8 teaspoon salt, pepper, and rosemary (if using). Recoat the skillet with nonstick cooking spray and place the chicken in the skillet, smooth side down. Cook for 3 minutes, turn, and add the mushrooms and wine.

EXCHANGES

3 Lean Meat

Calories 173
  Calories from Fat 50

Total Fat 6 g
  Saturated Fat 1 g

Cholesterol 66 mg

Sodium 248 mg

Total Carbohydrate 3 g
  Dietary Fiber 1 g
  Sugars 1 g

Protein 25 g

COOK'S TIP

Be sure to pat the
chicken very dry with
paper towels, or it won't
brown properly.

3 Bring the mixture to a boil, reduce the heat, cover tightly, and simmer 10 minutes or until the chicken is no longer pink in the center. Remove the chicken only, shaking off any mushrooms, and set it aside on a serving platter. Cover it with foil to keep warm.

4 Increase the heat to medium high, bring the mushroom mixture to a boil, and continue to boil 2–3 minutes or until most of the liquid has evaporated. Remove from the heat, stir in the margarine, and spoon over the chicken.

TANGY CHICKEN AND PEPPERS

Serves 4/Serving size: 2 drumsticks plus 1/2 cup peppers

PREP TIME: 15 MINUTES
COOK TIME: 42 MINUTES
STAND TIME: 5 MINUTES

8 chicken drumsticks, skin removed, rinsed and patted dry

1 large green bell pepper, thinly sliced

1 medium onion, thinly sliced

1 cup water

1/2 teaspoon salt (divided use)

1/8 teaspoon black pepper

1/4 cup ketchup

1. Place a large nonstick skillet over medium-high heat until hot. Coat the skillet with nonstick cooking spray, add the drumsticks, and cook 8 minutes or until the drumsticks begin to brown, turning occasionally. Set the drumsticks aside on a separate plate.

2. Recoat the skillet and pan residue with nonstick cooking spray and reduce the heat to medium. Add the peppers and onions and cook 3 minutes, or until they begin to lightly brown on the edges, stirring frequently.

3. Add the drumsticks and plate juices, water, 1/4 teaspoon salt, and pepper to the skillet. Increase the heat to high and bring to a boil. Reduce the heat, cover tightly, and simmer 30–35 minutes or until the drumsticks are no longer pink in the center, turning occasionally.

EXCHANGES

2 Vegetable
4 Lean Meat

Calories 268
  Calories from Fat 69
Total Fat 8 g
  Saturated Fat 2 g
Cholesterol 123 mg
Sodium 599 mg
Total Carbohydrate 10 g
  Dietary Fiber 2 g
  Sugars 4 g
Protein 38 g

COOK'S TIP

To skin the drumsticks easily and quickly, use one paper towel per drumstick. Grab the skin with the paper towel and pull. You'll get great traction and the chicken skin won't slip between your fingers!

4 Place the drumsticks in a shallow pasta bowl or rimmed serving platter. Add the ketchup and 1/4 teaspoon salt to the pepper mixture in the skillet. Increase the heat to high, bring to a boil, and continue boiling 1 minute or until the mixture is reduced to 2 cups.

5 Spoon the pepper mixture over the drumsticks, cover, and let stand 5 minutes to develop flavors.

CHILI'D TURKEY BREAST AU JUS

Serves 12/Serving size: 4 ounces

PREP TIME: 20 MINUTES
COOK TIME: 1 HOUR AND 45 MINUTES
STAND TIME: 20 MINUTES

1 1/2 teaspoons chili powder

3/4 teaspoon dried sage

1/2 teaspoon dried rosemary

1/2 teaspoon black pepper

3/4 teaspoon salt (divided use)

6-pound frozen turkey breast with bone in, thawed, rinsed, and patted dry

2/3 cup cold water

1. Preheat the oven to 325 degrees.

2. Stir the chili powder, sage, rosemary, pepper, and 1/2 teaspoon salt together in a small bowl until well blended. Loosen the skin on the turkey breast by sliding your fingertips between the skin and the turkey meat (do not remove skin). Rub the chili mixture on the turkey meat under the skin.

3. Coat a 13 × 9-inch baking rack and pan with nonstick cooking spray, place the turkey on the baking rack, and bake 1 hour and 45 minutes or until a meat thermometer reaches 165 degrees. Place the turkey on a cutting board and let stand 20 minutes.

EXCHANGES
4 Lean Meat

Calories 176
   Calories from Fat 9

Total Fat 1 g
   Saturated Fat 0 g

Cholesterol 107 mg

Sodium 216 mg

Total Carbohydrate 0 g
   Dietary Fiber 0 g
   Sugars 0 g

Protein 39 g

COOK'S TIP

If you use a zippered plastic bag to separate the grease, first pour the pan drippings into a 2-cup measuring cup, then into the bag. To remove the grease, hold the bag over a small glass bowl or saucepan, snip off a bottom corner of the bag, and allow the juice to run out, stopping when the grease is all that is left in the bag.

4 Meanwhile, add the water and remaining 1/4 teaspoon salt to the pan drippings and stir until well blended. Carefully pour the pan drippings into a grease separator or a plastic zippered bag. Freeze the drippings for 10 minutes to separate the grease.

5 Remove the grease from the separator or bag, pour into a glass dish, and heat in the microwave on HIGH for 30 seconds. Slice the turkey, discard the skin, and serve with the drippings.

HOISIN CHICKEN

Serves 4/Serving size: 3 ounces

PREP TIME: 10 MINUTES
COOK TIME: 8 MINUTES

3 tablespoons hoisin sauce

1 teaspoon orange zest

3 tablespoons orange juice

1 pound boneless, skinless chicken breasts, rinsed, patted dry, and cut into thin slices or strips

1 Stir the hoisin sauce, orange zest, and juice together in a small bowl and set aside.

2 Place a medium nonstick skillet over medium-high heat until hot. Coat the skillet with nonstick cooking spray, add the chicken, and cook 6–7 minutes or until the chicken just begins to lightly brown. Use two utensils to stir as you would when stir-frying.

3 Place the chicken on a serving platter. Add the hoisin mixture to the skillet and cook 15 seconds, stirring constantly. Spoon evenly over the chicken.

COOK'S TIP

For a striking contrast in color and flavor, serve on a bed of stir-fried snow peas or asparagus.

EXCHANGES

1/2 Carbohydrate
3 Lean Meat

Calories 152
  Calories from Fat 29

Total Fat 3 g
  Saturated Fat 1 g

Cholesterol 66 mg

Sodium 210 mg

Total Carbohydrate 5 g
  Dietary Fiber 0 g
  Sugars 5 g

Protein 25 g

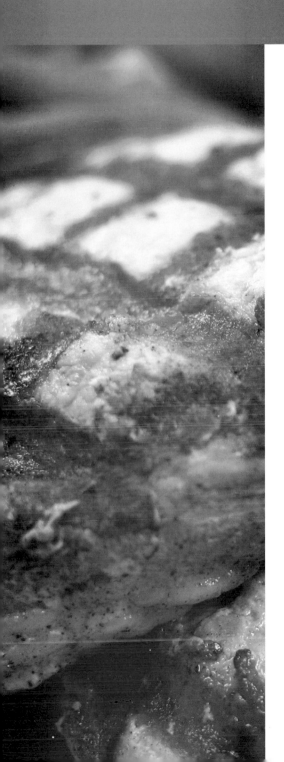

PORK

COUNTRY-STYLE HAM AND POTATO CASSEROLE

Serves 4/Serving size: 1 1/2 cups

PREP TIME: 15 MINUTES
BAKE TIME: 40–45 MINUTES
STAND TIME: 3 MINUTES

8 ounces lean smoked deli ham, (preferably Virginia ham), thinly sliced and chopped

1 pound red potatoes, scrubbed and thinly sliced

1 medium onion, thinly sliced

Black pepper to taste

1/3 cup shredded, reduced-fat, sharp cheddar cheese

1   Preheat the oven to 350 degrees.

2   Place a medium nonstick skillet over medium-high heat until hot. Coat the skillet with nonstick cooking spray, add ham, and cook 5 minutes or until the ham edges are beginning to lightly brown, stirring frequently. Remove from the heat and set the ham aside on a separate plate.

3   Layer half of the potatoes and half of the onions in the bottom of the skillet. Top with the ham and repeat with layers of potatoes and onions. Sprinkle with black pepper and cover tightly with a sheet of foil.

4   Bake 35–40 minutes or until the potatoes are tender when pierced with a fork. Remove from the oven, top with cheese, and let stand, uncovered, for 3 minutes to melt the cheese and develop flavors.

COOK'S TIP

Nonstick skillets will work fine in 350-degree temperatures, even with plastic handles. You may cover the handle with foil, if you like. Or use an 12 × 8-inch glass baking dish (but you'll miss the flavor added by the skillet drippings).

EXCHANGES

2 Starch
1 Lean Meat

Calories 202
  Calories from Fat 39

Total Fat 4 g
  Saturated Fat 2 g

Cholesterol 34 mg

Sodium 573 mg

Total Carbohydrate 28 g
  Dietary Fiber 2 g
  Sugars 4 g

Protein 15 g

SAUSAGE PILAF PEPPERS

Serves 4/Serving size: 1 pepper

PREP TIME: 8 MINUTES
COOK TIME: 40 MINUTES

4 medium green bell peppers

6 ounces 50% reduced-fat pork breakfast sausage

3/4 cup uncooked instant brown rice

2/3 cup salsa (divided use)

1 Preheat the oven to 350 degrees.

2 Slice the tops off of each pepper and discard the seeds and membrane, leaving the peppers whole.

3 Coat a large nonstick skillet with nonstick cooking spray and place over medium-high heat until hot. Add the sausage and cook until it's no longer pink, breaking up large pieces while stirring.

4 Remove from the heat and add the rice and all but 4 tablespoons salsa. Stir gently to blend.

5 Fill the peppers with equal amounts of the mixture and top each with 1 tablespoon salsa. Place the peppers in the skillet and cover tightly with foil. Bake 35 minutes or until the peppers are tender.

COOK'S TIP

Nonstick skillets will work fine in 350-degree temperatures, even with plastic handles. You may cover the handle with foil, if you like. Or use a small glass baking dish.

EXCHANGES

1 Starch
2 Vegetable
2 Fat

Calories 264
  Calories from Fat 90

Total Fat 10 g
  Saturated Fat 3 g

Cholesterol 29 mg

Sodium 540 mg

Total Carbohydrate 37 g
  Dietary Fiber 4 g
  Sugars 5 g

Protein 12 g

ANYTIME SKILLET PORK

Serves 4/Serving size: 1 chop

PREP TIME: 5 MINUTES
COOK TIME: 10 MINUTES

4 thin pork chops with bone in, trimmed of fat
(about 1 1/4 pounds total)

Black pepper to taste

1/3 cup water

1 1/2 teaspoons Worcestershire sauce

1 1/2 teaspoons lite soy sauce

1. Place a large nonstick skillet over medium-high heat until hot. Coat with nonstick cooking spray.

2. Liberally sprinkle the pork chops with pepper and cook 3 minutes. Turn and cook 3 more minutes or until the pork is barely pink in the center. Set the pork aside on a separate plate and cover with foil to keep warm.

3. Stir the remaining ingredients together in a small bowl. Add the mixture to the skillet and bring to a boil over medium-high heat. Boil for 3–4 minutes or until the liquid is reduced to 2 tablespoons, stirring frequently. Spoon the sauce over the pork.

COOK'S TIP

Try this for breakfast on a cold wintry day!

EXCHANGES

3 Lean Meat

Calories 144
    Calories from Fat 52

Total Fat 6 g
    Saturated Fat 2 g

Cholesterol 59 mg

Sodium 139 mg

Total Carbohydrate 1 g
    Dietary Fiber 0 g
    Sugars 0 g

Protein 21 g

COOK'S TIP

Don't overcook the pork chops in Step 3—they continue to cook while you finish the dish.

EXCHANGES

3 Lean Meat

Calories 162
   Calories from Fat 65
Total Fat 7 g
   Saturated Fat 3 g
Cholesterol 58 mg
Sodium 255 mg
Total Carbohydrate 2 g
   Dietary Fiber 1 g
   Sugars 0 g
Protein 21 g

PORK WITH TOMATO–CAPER SAUCE

Serves 4/Serving size: 1 chop

PREP TIME: 10 MINUTES
COOK TIME: 10 MINUTES

2 tablespoons tomato paste with oregano, basil, and garlic

2 tablespoons capers, drained and mashed with a fork

2/3 cup water (divided use)

1/8 teaspoon salt

4 4-ounce boneless pork chops, trimmed of fat

1 Using a fork, stir the tomato paste, capers, and 1/3 cup water together in a small bowl.

2 Place a medium nonstick skillet over medium-high heat until hot. Coat the skillet with nonstick cooking spray, add the pork chops, and cook 3 minutes.

3 Turn the pork chops and immediately reduce the heat to medium. Spoon the tomato mixture evenly on top of each pork chop, cover tightly, and cook 5 minutes or until the pork chops are barely pink in the center. The sauce may be dark in some areas.

4 Remove the skillet from the heat and add the remaining 1/3 cup water and salt. Turn the pork chops over several times to remove the sauce. Place the pork chops on a serving plate and set aside.

5 Increase the heat to medium high. Bring the sauce to a boil, stirring constantly, and boil 1 minute or until the sauce begins to thicken slightly and measures 1/2 cup. Spoon the sauce over the pork chops.

PORK WITH PINEAPPLE–GINGER SALSA

Serves 4/Serving size: 1 chop plus 1/4 cup salsa

PREP TIME: 10 MINUTES
COOK TIME: 12 MINUTES

8-ounce can pineapple tidbits packed in juice, drained, reserve juice

2 teaspoons grated gingerroot

1/2–1 medium jalapeño, seeded and minced

1 teaspoon pourable sugar substitute (optional)

4 4-ounce boneless pork chops, trimmed of fat

1/4 teaspoon salt

1/4 teaspoon black pepper

1 Stir the pineapple, 1 tablespoon of the reserved pineapple juice, gingerroot, jalapeño, and sugar substitute (if using), together in a small bowl and set aside.

2 Sprinkle both sides of the pork evenly with salt and pepper.

3 Place a large nonstick skillet over medium-high heat until hot. Coat the skillet with nonstick cooking spray, add the pork, and cook 4 minutes. Turn and cook 4 minutes longer or until the pork is barely pink in the center.

4 Add the remaining pineapple juice to the pork in the skillet and cook 2 minutes. Turn and cook 1 minute longer or until the liquid has evaporated. Remove the skillet from the heat, turn the pork several times to lightly glaze with the salsa, and serve.

COOK'S TIP

If tidbits are not available, use pineapple chunks and cut them in smaller pieces.

EXCHANGES
1/2 Fruit
2 Lean Meat

Calories 155
  Calories from Fat 27
Total Fat 3 g
  Saturated Fat 1 g
Cholesterol 0 mg
Sodium 187 mg
Total Carbohydrate 10 g
  Dietary Fiber 1 g
  Sugars 9 g
Protein 22 g

GRAPEFRUIT-ZESTED PORK

Serves 4/Serving size: 1 chop

PREP TIME: 8 MINUTES
MARINATE TIME: 8 HOURS
COOK TIME: 6 MINUTES

3 tablespoons lite soy sauce

1/2–1 teaspoon grapefruit zest

3 tablespoons grapefruit juice

1 jalapeño pepper, seeded and finely chopped,
or 1/8–1/4 teaspoon dried red pepper flakes

4 thin pork chops with bone in (about 1 1/4 pounds total)

1 Combine all ingredients in a large zippered plastic bag. Seal tightly and toss back and forth to coat evenly. Refrigerate overnight or at least 8 hours.

2 Preheat the broiler.

3 Coat the broiler rack and pan with nonstick cooking spray, arrange the pork chops on the rack (discarding the marinade), and broil 2 inches away from the heat source for 3 minutes. Turn and broil 3 minutes longer or until the pork is no longer pink in the center.

COOK'S TIP

You can marinate the pork up to 48 hours, if you like.

EXCHANGES

3 Lean Meat

Calories 161
 Calories from Fat 52

Total Fat 6 g
 Saturated Fat 2 g

Cholesterol 59 mg

Sodium 259 mg

Total Carbohydrate 4 g
 Dietary Fiber 0 g
 Sugars 3 g

Protein 22 g

SWEET SHERRY'D PORK TENDERLOIN

Serves 4/Serving size: 3 ounces pork plus 2 tablespoons sauce

PREP TIME: 4 MINUTES
MARINATE TIME: 8 HOURS
COOK TIME: 22 MINUTES
STAND TIME: 3 MINUTES

1 pound pork tenderloin

1/4 cup dry sherry (divided use)

3 tablespoons lite soy sauce (divided use)

1/3 cup peach all-fruit spread

Black pepper to taste

1 Place the pork, 2 tablespoons sherry, and 2 tablespoons soy sauce in a quart-sized zippered plastic bag. Seal tightly and toss back and forth to coat evenly. Refrigerate overnight or at least 8 hours.

2 Stir the fruit spread, 2 tablespoons sherry, and 1 tablespoon soy sauce together in a small bowl. Cover with plastic wrap and refrigerate until needed.

3 Preheat the oven to 425 degrees.

4 Remove the pork from the marinade and discard the marinade. Place a medium nonstick skillet over medium-high heat until hot. Coat the skillet with nonstick cooking spray, add the pork, and brown on all sides.

EXCHANGES

1 Carbohydrate
3 Lean Meat

Calories 186
  Calories from Fat 26

Total Fat 3 g
  Saturated Fat 1 g

Cholesterol 61 mg

Sodium 334 mg

Total Carbohydrate 15 g
  Dietary Fiber 0 g
  Sugars 12 g

Protein 23 g

5 Place the pork in a 9-inch pie pan and bake 15 minutes or until the pork is barely pink in the center. Place the pork on a cutting board and let stand 3 minutes before slicing.

6 Meanwhile, place the fruit spread mixture in the skillet and bring to a boil over medium-high heat, stirring frequently. Place the sauce on the bottom of a serving plate and arrange the pork on top. Sprinkle evenly with black pepper.

COOK'S TIP

You can marinate the
pork up to 48 hours,
if you like.

SWEET JERK PORK

Serves 4/Serving size: 3 ounces

PREP TIME: 7 MINUTES
MARINATE TIME: 15 MINUTES
COOK TIME: 20 MINUTES
STAND TIME: 25 MINUTES

1 pound pork tenderloin

2 teaspoons jerk seasoning

2 tablespoons packed dark brown sugar

2 teaspoons Worcestershire sauce

1 Preheat the oven to 425 degrees.

2 Sprinkle the pork evenly with the jerk seasoning and press down gently so the spices adhere. Let the pork stand 15 minutes.

3 Stir the sugar and Worcestershire sauce together in a small bowl until well blended. Coat an 11 × 7-inch baking pan with nonstick cooking spray and set aside.

4 Place a large nonstick skillet over medium-high heat until hot. Coat the skillet with nonstick cooking spray, add the pork, and brown all sides, about 5 minutes, turning occasionally.

5 Place the pork in the baking pan and spoon all but 1 tablespoon of the Worcestershire mixture evenly over the pork. Bake for 13–15 minutes or until the pork is barely pink in the center and a meat thermometer reaches 170 degrees.

6 Place the pork on a cutting board, spoon the remaining 1 tablespoon Worcestershire mixture evenly over all, and let stand 10 minutes before slicing.

COOK'S TIP

Since pork tenderloins are usually sold in 2-pound packages, 2 tenderloins to a package, use one in this recipe and wrap the other one in plastic wrap and freeze for another use.

EXCHANGES

1/2 Carbohydrate
3 Lean Meat

Calories 150
    Calories from Fat 26

Total Fat 3 g
    Saturated Fat 1 g

Cholesterol 61 mg

Sodium 216 mg

Total Carbohydrate 8 g
    Dietary Fiber 0 g
    Sugars 8 g

Protein 22 g

PORK WITH KALAMATA RICE

Serves 4/Serving size: 3 ounces pork plus 1/2 cup rice

PREP TIME: 9 MINUTES
COOK TIME: 8 MINUTES

1/3 cup medium salsa

12 small kalamata olives, pitted and coarsely chopped

2 cups cooked brown rice, warm (omit added salt or fat)

4 4-ounce boneless pork chops, trimmed of fat

1/4 teaspoon salt

1/4 teaspoon black pepper

1/2 cup water

1 Add the salsa and olives to the cooked rice and toss gently. Place on a serving platter and cover with a sheet of foil to keep warm.

2 Place a large nonstick skillet over medium-high heat until hot. Coat the skillet with nonstick cooking spray. Sprinkle the pork with salt and pepper. Place the pork in the skillet, immediately reduce the heat to medium, and cook 4 minutes. Turn and cook 4 minutes longer or until the pork is barely pink in the center. Place the pork on top of the rice, cover with foil, and set aside.

3 Add the water to the skillet, stir, and bring to a boil over medium-high heat. Boil 2 minutes or until the liquid is reduced to 1/4 cup. Pour the sauce over the pork and rice.

COOK'S TIP

Adding the water to the pan drippings (a cooking technique called deglazing) in the last step pulls the flavors together while adding moisture to the dish.

EXCHANGES

1 1/2 Starch
3 Lean Meat

Calories 279
  Calories from Fat 82

Total Fat 9 g
  Saturated Fat 3 g

Cholesterol 58 mg

Sodium 409 mg

Total Carbohydrate 24 g
  Dietary Fiber 2 g
  Sugars 1 g

Protein 24 g

SIZZLING PORK CHOPS

Serves 4/Serving size: 1 chop

PREP TIME: 3 MINUTES
COOK TIME: 12 MINUTES
STAND TIME: 2 MINUTES

4 4-ounce boneless pork chops, trimmed of fat

1 tablespoon dried zesty Italian salad dressing and recipe mix (available in packets)

1 Coat both sides of the pork chops with the salad dressing mix, pressing down gently so the spices adhere.

2 Place a large nonstick skillet over medium heat until hot. Coat the skillet with nonstick cooking spray, add the pork, and cook 4 minutes. Turn and cook 4 minutes longer or until the pork is barely pink in the center.

3 Remove the skillet from the heat and let the pork stand in the skillet 2–3 minutes or until the pork begins to release some of its juices. Move the pork pieces around in the skillet several times to absorb the pan residue.

COOK'S TIP

Allowing the pork chops to stand briefly in the skillet, then moving them around in the pan, gives them a deep, dark color and rich flavor without adding other high-fat ingredients.

EXCHANGES

3 Lean Meat

Calories 159
  Calories from Fat 64
Total Fat 7 g
  Saturated Fat 3 g
Cholesterol 58 mg
Sodium 383 mg
Total Carbohydrate 1 g
  Dietary Fiber 0 g
  Sugars 1 g
Protein 21 g

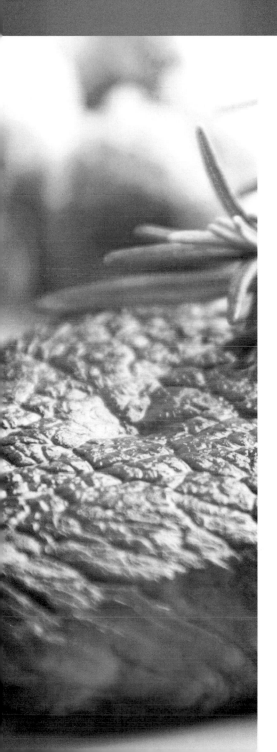

BEEF

HOMESTYLE DOUBLE-ONION ROAST

Serves 6/Serving size: 3 1/2 ounces beef plus 2/3 cup vegetables

PREP TIME: 20 MINUTES
COOK TIME: 1 HOUR AND 10 MINUTES
STAND TIME: 15 MINUTES

1 pound carrots, scrubbed, quartered lengthwise, and cut into 3-inch pieces

2 medium onions (8 ounces total), cut in 1/2-inch wedges and separated

1 3/4 pound lean eye of round roast

1/4 cup water

1-ounce packet onion soup mix

1 Preheat the oven to 325 degrees.

2 Coat a 13 × 9-inch nonstick baking pan with nonstick cooking spray, arrange the carrots and onions in the pan, and set aside.

3 Place a medium nonstick skillet over medium-high heat until hot. Coat the skillet with nonstick cooking spray, add the beef, and brown 2 minutes. Turn and brown another 2 minutes.

4 Place the beef in the center of the baking pan on top of the vegetables. Add the water to the skillet and scrap up the pan drippings, then pour them over the beef. Sprinkle evenly with the soup mix.

EXCHANGES

2 Vegetable
3 Lean Meat

Calories 229
  Calories from Fat 43

Total Fat 5 g
  Saturated Fat 2 g

Cholesterol 58 mg

Sodium 541 mg

Total Carbohydrate 13 g
  Dietary Fiber 3 g
  Sugars 7 g

Protein 32 g

COOK'S TIP

These leftovers freeze
well for later use.

5 Cover the pan tightly with foil and cook 1 hour and 5 minutes or until a meat thermometer reaches 135 degrees. Place the beef on a cutting board and let stand 15 minutes before slicing. (The temperature will rise another 10 degrees while the beef stands.)

6 Keep the vegetables in the pan covered to keep warm. Place the beef slices on a serving platter, arrange the vegetables around the beef, and spoon the pan liquids evenly over the beef.

SIMPLY SEARED BEEF TENDERLOIN

Serves 4/Serving size: 1 steak

PREP TIME: 3 MINUTES
COOK TIME: 11 MINUTES

4 5-ounce beef tenderloin steaks, about 3/4-inch thick, trimmed of fat

1 large split garlic clove

1/4 teaspoon coarsely ground black pepper

1/4 teaspoon salt

2 teaspoons Worcestershire sauce

1/2 teaspoon beef bouillon granules

1/2 cup water

1   Rub the beef with the garlic clove. Place a large non-stick skillet over medium-high heat until hot. Coat the skillet with nonstick cooking spray, add the beef, and cook 3 minutes. Turn and cook another 2 minutes.

2   Reduce the heat to medium low and cook the steaks 4 minutes longer or until they are done as desired, turning once. Set aside on a separate plate.

3   Increase the heat to medium high, add the remaining ingredients, bring to a boil, and continue boiling 1 minute or until the mixture measures 1/4 cup liquid. Pour the juices over the beef.

COOK'S TIP

You can also prepare this beef with 1/2 cup strong coffee instead of the bouillon granules and water—you'll find the coffee intensifies the hearty beef flavor.

EXCHANGES

3 Lean Meat

Calories 180
    Calories from Fat 65

Total Fat 7 g
    Saturated Fat 3 g

Cholesterol 72 mg

Sodium 344 mg

Total Carbohydrate 1 g
    Dietary Fiber 0 g
    Sugars 1 g

Protein 26 g

COOK'S TIP

To grate fresh gingerroot, first peel off the outer skin with a sharp knife and use a fine grater for best results.

EXCHANGES

4 Lean Meat

Calories 244
  Calories from Fat 51

Total Fat 6 g
  Saturated Fat 2 g

Cholesterol 102 mg

Sodium 338 mg

Total Carbohydrate 4 g
  Dietary Fiber 0 g
  Sugars 4 g

Protein 42 g

BEEF STRIPS WITH SWEET GINGER SAUCE

Serves 4/Serving size: 1/2 cup

PREP TIME: 4 MINUTES
COOK TIME: 4 MINUTES

2 tablespoons lite soy sauce

1 tablespoon sugar

2 teaspoons grated gingerroot

1 pound boneless top round or sirloin steak, trimmed of fat and sliced into strips

1 Stir the soy sauce, sugar, and gingerroot together in a small bowl and set aside.

2 Place a large nonstick skillet over medium high until hot. Coat the skillet with nonstick cooking spray, add half the beef, and cook 1 minute, stirring constantly.

3 Remove the beef from the skillet and set aside on a separate plate. Recoat the skillet with nonstick cooking spray and cook the remaining beef 1 minute.

4 Return the first batch of beef to the skillet, add the soy sauce mixture, and cook 1 minute to heat thoroughly.

SIRLOIN HOAGIES

Serves 4/Serving size: 1 hoagie

PREP TIME: 12 MINUTES
COOK TIME: 16 MINUTES

1/4 teaspoon salt (divided use)

1/2 teaspoon black pepper

1 pound boneless sirloin steak, trimmed of fat

1 large onion, thinly sliced (about 1 1/2 cups)

1/2 cup water

8 ounces whole wheat or white French bread

1 1/2 tablespoons prepared mustard

1 Preheat the oven to 350 degrees.

2 Sprinkle 1/8 teaspoon salt and the pepper evenly over both sides of the steak. Place a large nonstick skillet over medium-high heat until hot. Coat the skillet with nonstick cooking spray, add the steak, and cook 5 minutes.

3 Turn and cook another 4 minutes or until the beef is done as desired. Place the beef on a cutting board and set aside.

4 Coat the pan drippings with nonstick cooking spray, reduce the heat to medium, and add the onions. Coat the onions with nonstick cooking spray and cook 6–7 minutes or until they are richly browned, stirring frequently.

5 Add the water to the onions and cook 1 minute or until most of the moisture has evaporated, stirring constantly. Remove from the heat.

EXCHANGES

2 Starch
1 Vegetable
3 Lean Meat

Calories 317
  Calories from Fat 55

Total Fat 6 g
  Saturated Fat 2 g

Cholesterol 42 mg

Sodium 602 mg

Total Carbohydrate 36 g
  Dietary Fiber 3 g
  Sugars 3 g

Protein 28 g

COOK'S TIP

When buying boneless beef or pork for a recipe asking you to trim the fat, purchase about 4 ounces more than the recipe calls for. For example, 1 1/4 pounds boneless beef or pork will yield 1 pound meat after you trim the fat.

6 Wrap the bread in foil, place it in the oven, and bake 5 minutes or until hot. Meanwhile, thinly slice the beef diagonally.

7 Using a serrated knife, cut the bread in half lengthwise and spread a thin layer of mustard on each cut side. Top with the beef, then onions and any juices. Sprinkle the beef with the remaining salt, top with the other bread half, and cut in fourths crosswise.

ZESTY BEEF PATTIES WITH GRILLED ONIONS

Serves 4/Serving size: 1 patty plus 1/4 cup onions

PREP TIME: 7 MINUTES
COOK TIME: 15 MINUTES

1 pound 90% lean ground beef

1 tablespoon Dijon mustard

2 tablespoons Ranch-style salad dressing and seasoning mix (available in packets)

1 large yellow onion, thinly sliced

1/4 cup water

1 Mix the ground beef, mustard, and salad dressing mix together in a medium bowl. Shape the beef mixture into 4 patties.

2 Place a large nonstick skillet over medium-high heat until hot. Coat the skillet with nonstick cooking spray and add the onions. Coat the onions with nonstick cooking spray and cook 7 minutes or until they are richly browned, stirring frequently. Set them aside on a separate plate.

3 Recoat the skillet with nonstick cooking spray, add the patties, and cook 4 minutes. Flip the patties and cook another 3 minutes or until they are no longer pink in the center. Place them on a serving platter.

4 Add the onions and water to the pan drippings and cook 30 seconds, scraping the bottom and sides of the skillet. When the mixture has thickened slightly, spoon it over the patties.

COOK'S TIP

Be sure to use the dry seasoning mix in this recipe, not the liquid Ranch dressing.

EXCHANGES

1 Vegetable
3 Lean Meat

Calories 215
  Calories from Fat 85

Total Fat 9 g
  Saturated Fat 4 g

Cholesterol 69 mg

Sodium 419 mg

Total Carbohydrate 8 g
  Dietary Fiber 1 g
  Sugars 3 g

Protein 23 g

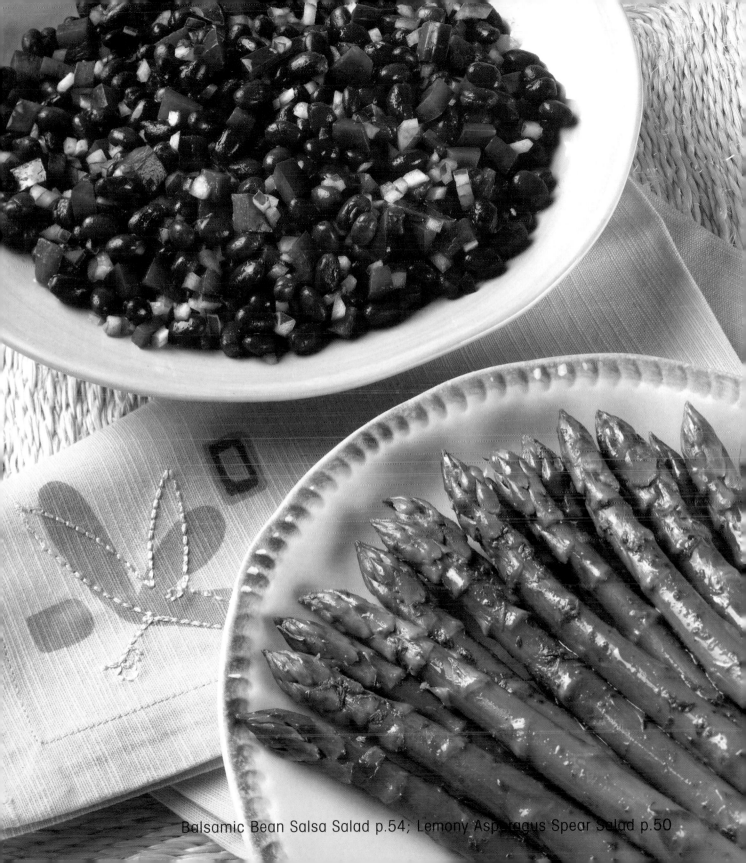

Balsamic Bean Salsa Salad p.54; Lemony Asparagus Spear Salad p.50

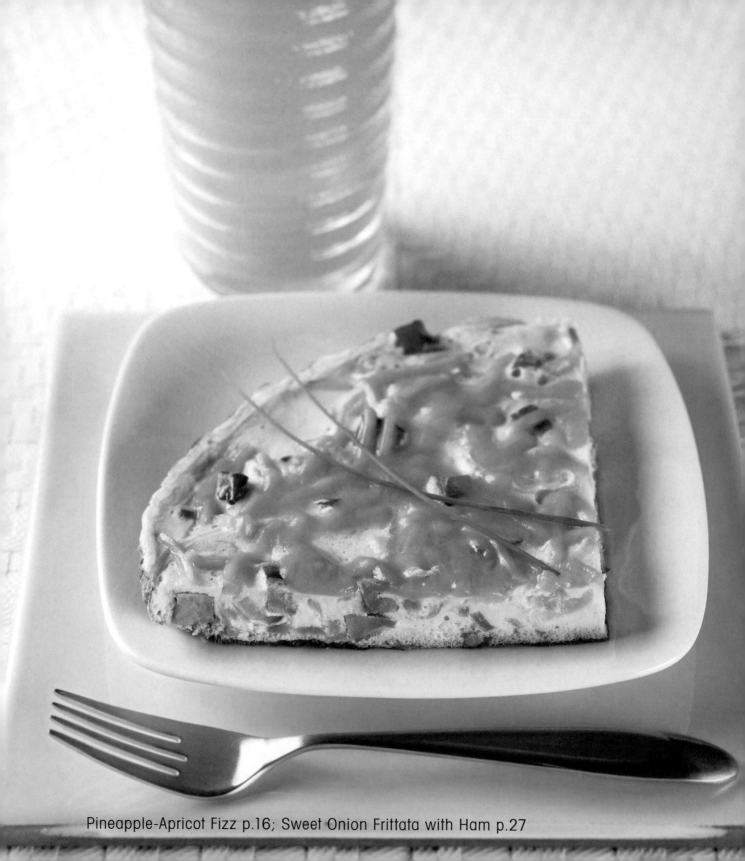

Pineapple-Apricot Fizz p.16; Sweet Onion Frittata with Ham p.27

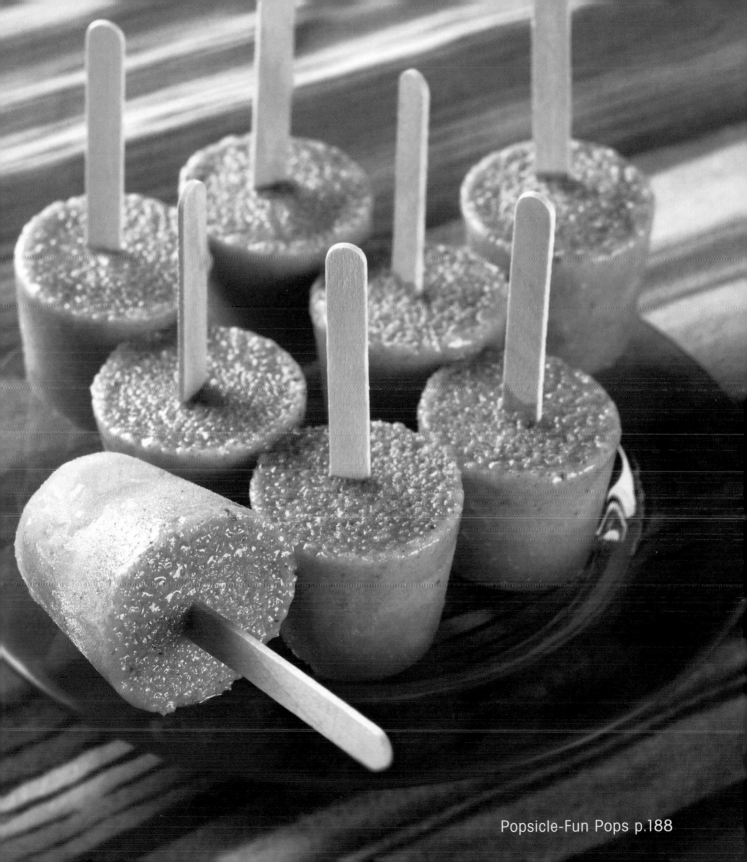

Popsicle-Fun Pops p.188

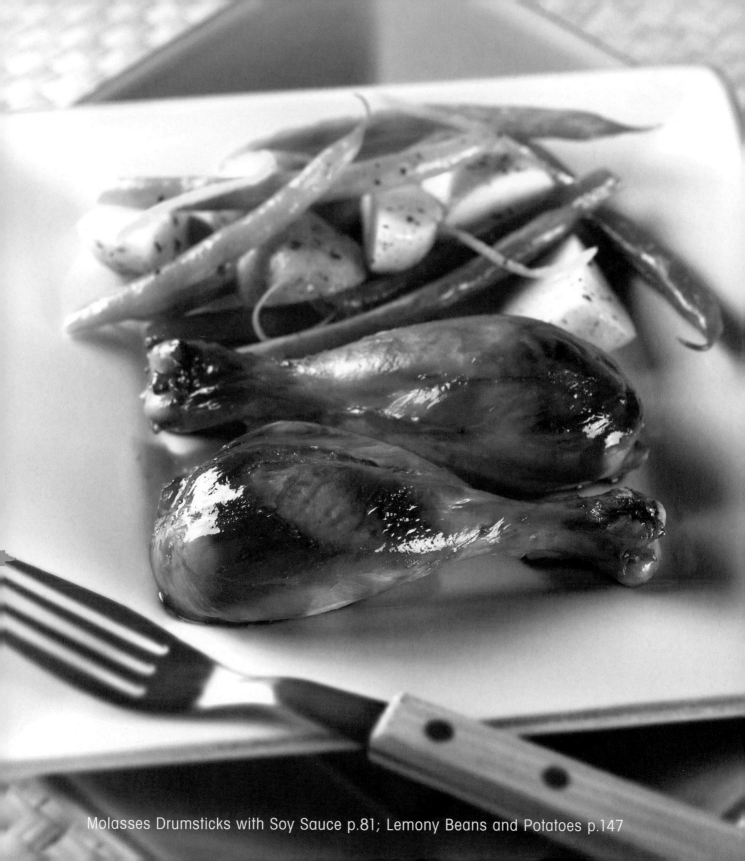

Molasses Drumsticks with Soy Sauce p.81; Lemony Beans and Potatoes p.147

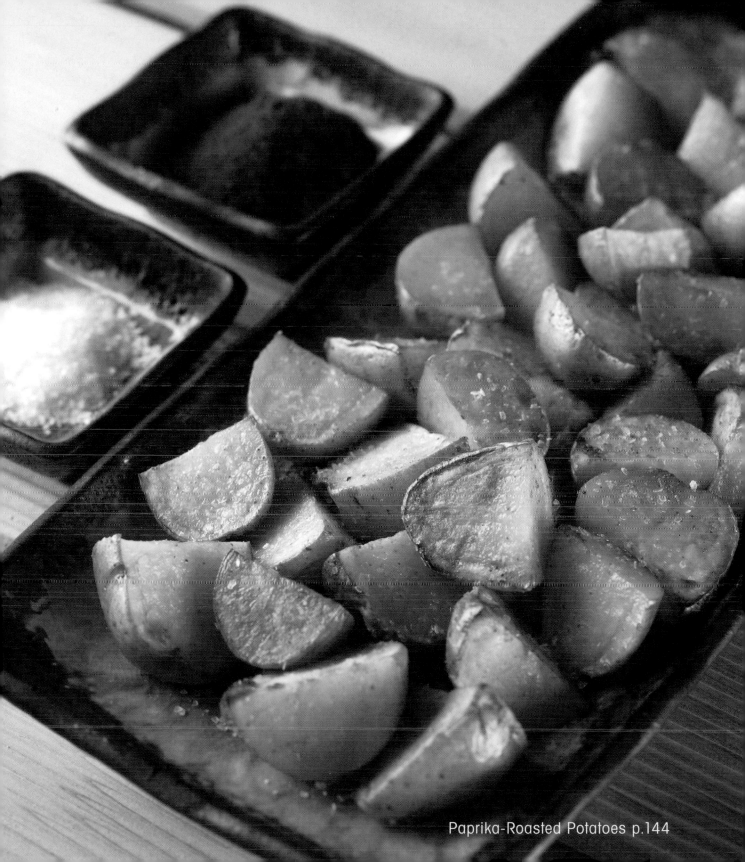

Paprika-Roasted Potatoes p.144

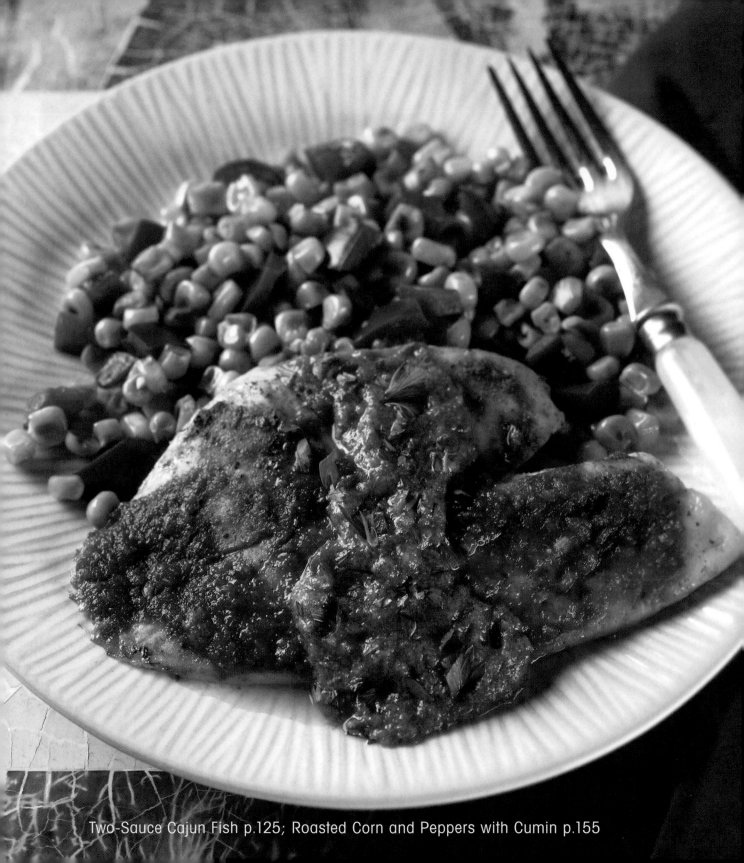
Two-Sauce Cajun Fish p.125; Roasted Corn and Peppers with Cumin p.155

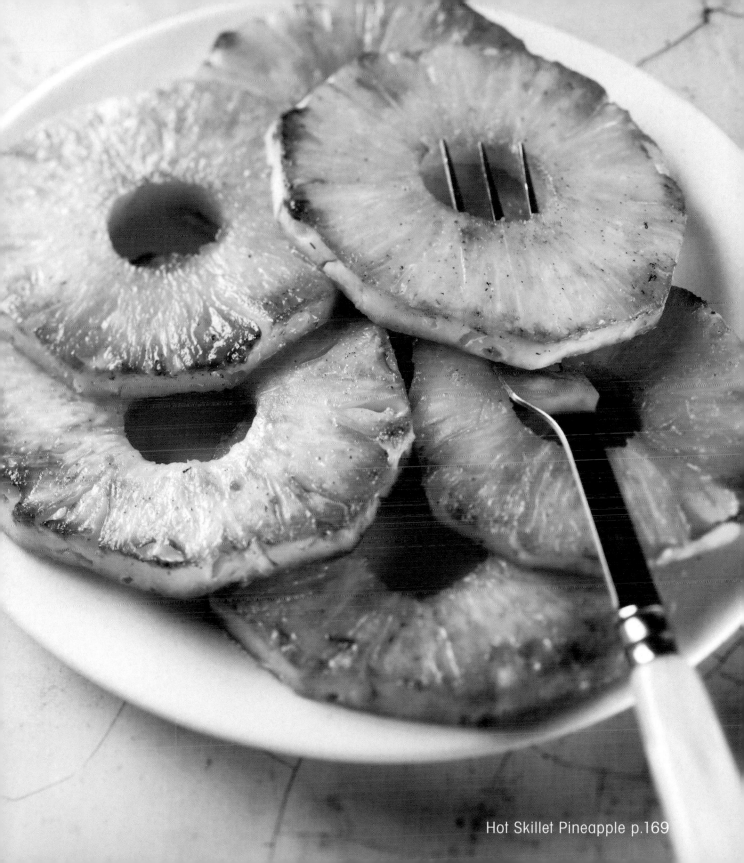

Hot Skillet Pineapple p.169

Fresh Berry and Cream Mini Tarts p.193; Light Raspberry Chocolate Cake p.187

CUMIN'D BEEF PATTIES AND SANTA FE SOUR CREAM

Serves 4/Serving size: 1 patty plus 1 1/2 tablespoons sour cream

PREP TIME: 5 MINUTES
COOK TIME: 8 MINUTES

1 pound 90% lean ground beef

1/3 cup mild picante sauce (divided use)

2 teaspoons ground cumin

1/4 teaspoon salt (divided use)

1/8 teaspoon black pepper

1/4 cup fat-free sour cream

1. Mix the ground beef, all but 2 tablespoons of the picante sauce, cumin, 1/8 teaspoon salt, and black pepper in a medium bowl until well blended. Shape the beef mixture into 4 patties.

2. Place a large nonstick skillet over medium-high heat until hot. Coat the skillet with nonstick cooking spray, add the patties, and cook 4 minutes. Flip the patties and cook another 3 minutes or until they are no longer pink in the center.

3. Meanwhile, stir 2 tablespoons picante sauce, 1/8 teaspoon salt, and the sour cream together in a small bowl.

4. Top each patty with 1 1/2 tablespoons sour cream. Spoon an additional 1/2 teaspoon picante sauce on top of each serving, if desired.

COOK'S TIP

Picante sauce is a bit thinner than salsa, but the two can be used interchangeably in most recipes.

EXCHANGES

3 Lean Meat

Calories 200
  Calories from Fat 86

Total Fat 10 g
  Saturated Fat 4 g

Cholesterol 70 mg

Sodium 390 mg

Total Carbohydrate 2 g
  Dietary Fiber 0 g
  Sugars 1 g

Protein 23 g

CHILI-STUFFED POTATOES

Serves 4/Serving size: 1 potato stuffed with 1/2 cup chili

PREP TIME: 5 MINUTES
COOK TIME: 10 MINUTES

4 8-ounce baking potatoes, preferably Yukon Gold, scrubbed and pierced several times with a fork

12 ounces 90% lean ground beef

3/4 cup water

1.25-ounce packet chili seasoning mix

1/4 teaspoon salt

1/2 cup reduced-fat sour cream or 1/3 cup shredded, reduced-fat, sharp cheddar cheese (optional)

1. Microwave the potatoes on HIGH 10–11 minutes or until they are tender when pierced with a fork.

2. Meanwhile, place a large nonstick skillet over medium-high heat until hot. Coat the skillet with nonstick cooking spray, add the beef, and cook until the beef is no longer pink, stirring frequently.

3. Add the water and chili seasoning and stir. Cook 1–2 minutes or until thickened.

4. Split the potatoes almost in half and fluff with a fork. Spoon 1/2 cup chili onto each potato and top with sour cream or cheese (if using).

COOK'S TIP

It's important to pierce the potatoes several times in different areas before microwaving them. This allows the built-up steam to be released and the potatoes to cook quicker.

EXCHANGES

3 Starch
2 Lean Meat

Calories 333
  Calories from Fat 69

Total Fat 8 g
  Saturated Fat 3 g

Cholesterol 51 mg

Sodium 517 mg

Total Carbohydrate 44 g
  Dietary Fiber 6 g
  Sugars 3 g

Protein 22 g

BOURBON'D FILET MIGNON

Serves 4/Serving size: 1 steak

PREP TIME: 5 MINUTES
MARINATE TIME: 15 MINUTES
COOK TIME: 8–12 MINUTES

1/2 teaspoon salt (divided use)

1/8–1/4 teaspoon coarsely ground black pepper

4 5-ounce filet mignon steaks (or beef tenderloin), about 3/4 inch thick, trimmed of fat

1/2 cup strong coffee (or 1/2 cup water and 1 teaspoon instant coffee granules)

2 tablespoons bourbon

2 teaspoons Worcestershire sauce

1   Sprinkle 1/4 teaspoon salt and black pepper evenly over both sides of the beef and let stand 15 minutes. Preheat the oven to 200 degrees.

2   Meanwhile, stir the coffee, bourbon, Worcestershire sauce, and 1/4 teaspoon salt together in a small bowl.

3   Place a large nonstick skillet over high heat until hot. Coat the skillet with nonstick cooking spray, add the steaks, and cook 3 minutes on each side.

4   Reduce the heat to medium low and cook the steaks 2–6 minutes longer or until they are done as desired. Place them on individual dinner plates in the oven.

5   Add the coffee mixture to the skillet, bring to a boil over high heat, and boil 2 minutes or until the liquid is reduced to 2 tablespoons. Spoon the sauce evenly over beef and serve immediately.

COOK'S TIP

There's no need to heat the water before combining it with the instant coffee granules. The granules dissolve just fine in cold water.

EXCHANGES

4 Lean Meat

Calories 195
  Calories from Fat 65

Total Fat 7 g
  Saturated Fat 3 g

Cholesterol 0 mg

Sodium 378 mg

Total Carbohydrate 1 g
  Dietary Fiber 0 g
  Sugars 1 g

Protein 26 g

STEWED BEEF AND ALE

Serves 4/Serving size: 3/4 cup

PREP TIME: 15 MINUTES
COOK TIME: 1 HOUR AND 40 MINUTES

1 pound boneless top round steak,
cut in 1/4 inch × 3 1/2 inch-strips

1 cup chopped onion

14.5-ounce can stewed tomatoes

1 cup beer

1 teaspoon sugar (optional)

1/4 teaspoon salt

1/4 teaspoon black pepper

1   Place a large nonstick skillet over medium-high heat
    until hot. Coat the skillet with nonstick cooking spray.
Working in two batches, add half of the beef strips and
brown, stirring constantly, and set aside on a separate
plate. Repeat with the remaining beef strips.

2   Recoat the skillet with nonstick cooking spray, add the
    onions, and cook 4 minutes or until the onions are
translucent, stirring frequently. Add the remaining ingredients, including the beef and any accumulated juices.

3   Bring to a boil over high heat, then reduce the heat,
    cover tightly, and simmer 1 hour and 30 minutes or
until the beef is very tender. Using the back of a spoon,
mash the beef pieces to thicken the dish slightly.

COOK'S TIP

You probably don't want
to omit the sugar in this
recipe—it offsets the
beer and calms down the
acidity of the tomatoes
(even though they are the
stewed variety, already a
little sweeter than other
canned tomatoes).

EXCHANGES

3 Vegetable
2 Lean Meat

Calories 183
    Calories from Fat 31
Total Fat 3 g
    Saturated Fat 1 g
Cholesterol 59 mg
Sodium 441 mg
Total Carbohydrate 13 g
    Dietary Fiber 2 g
    Sugars 6 g
Protein 25 g

COOK'S TIP

This recipe makes
a great meatball
sandwich.

EXCHANGES

1 1/2 Carbohydrate
3 Lean Meat

Calories 278
  Calories from Fat 90

Total Fat 10 g
  Saturated Fat 3 g

Cholesterol 46 mg

Sodium 698 mg

Total Carbohydrate 22 g
  Dietary Fiber 3 g
  Sugars 13 g

Protein 20 g

EXTRA EASY MEATBALLS

Serves 6/Serving size: 2/3 cup (4 meatballs plus sauce)

PREP TIME: 15 MINUTES
COOK TIME: 30 MINUTES

1 pound 90% lean ground beef

1/2 cup quick-cooking oats

3 large egg whites

1 tablespoon dried basil (optional)

26.5-ounce jar meatless spaghetti sauce (divided use)

1 Mix the ground beef, oats, egg whites, basil, and 1/2 cup spaghetti sauce together in a large bowl. Shape the mixture into 24 1-inch meatballs.

2 Place a large nonstick skillet over medium-high heat until hot. Coat with nonstick cooking spray, add the meatballs, and cook until browned, stirring frequently. Use two utensils to stir as you would when stir-frying.

3 Add the remaining spaghetti sauce and bring just to a boil. Reduce the heat, cover tightly, and simmer 20 minutes.

TENDER GREEN PEPPER'D TOP ROUND

Serves 4/Serving size: 1/4 recipe

PREP TIME: 10 MINUTES
MARINATE TIME: 8 HOURS
COOK TIME: 60 MINUTES

1 pound boneless top round steak, trimmed of fat and cut in 4 equal pieces

1/4 cup fat-free Italian salad dressing

1 cup water

1/4 cup ketchup

1/2 teaspoon salt

1/4 teaspoon black pepper

2 medium green bell peppers, cut in thin strips

1 Place the beef and salad dressing in a large zippered plastic bag. Seal tightly and shake back and forth to coat evenly. Refrigerate overnight or at least 8 hours, turning occasionally.

2 Stir the water, ketchup, salt, and black pepper together in a small bowl and set aside.

3 Place a large nonstick skillet over medium-high heat until hot. Coat the skillet with nonstick cooking spray. Remove the beef from the marinade, discard the marinade, and place the steaks in the skillet. Cook 3 minutes, then turn and cook another 2 minutes.

4 Reduce the heat to medium low and cook the steaks 4 minutes longer or until they are done as desired, turning once. Add the green peppers and pour the ketchup mixture over all. Bring to a boil, reduce the heat, cover tightly, and simmer 55 minutes or until very tender.

COOK'S TIP

Here's a great timesaver: buy an extra pound of steak, place it in a zippered plastic bag with 1/4 cup Italian salad dressing, and freeze it for a later use. It will marinate while freezing and defrosting, and you can have flavorful meat in a flash!

EXCHANGES

1/2 Carbohydrate
3 Lean Meat

Calories 167
    Calories from Fat 31
Total Fat 3 g
    Saturated Fat 1 g
Cholesterol 59 mg
Sodium 617 mg
Total Carbohydrate 9 g
    Dietary Fiber 1 g
    Sugars 5 g
Protein 24 g

SPICY CHILI'D SIRLOIN STEAK

Serves 4/Serving size: 3 ounces

PREP TIME: 2 MINUTES
MARINATE TIME: 15 MINUTES
COOK TIME: 11 MINUTES
STAND TIME: 2 MINUTES

1 pound boneless sirloin steak, trimmed of fat

2 tablespoons chili seasoning (available in packets)

1/8 teaspoon salt

1. Coat both sides of the sirloin with the chili seasoning mix, pressing down so the spices adhere. Let stand 15 minutes, or overnight in the refrigerator for a spicier flavor (let steak stand at room temperature 15 minutes before cooking).

2. Place a large nonstick skillet over medium-high heat until hot. Coat the skillet with nonstick cooking spray, add the beef, and cook 5 minutes. Turn the steak, reduce the heat to medium, cover tightly, and cook 5 minutes. Do not overcook. Remove the skillet from the heat and let stand 2 minutes, covered.

3. Sprinkle the steak with salt and cut into 1/4-inch slices. Pour any accumulated juices over the steak slices.

COOK'S TIP

Cooking the steak quickly at a higher temperature, then reducing the heat and covering the skillet, sears in the delicious meat juices without drying out the meat.

EXCHANGES

3 Lean Meat

Calories 148
  Calories from Fat 40

Total Fat 4 g
  Saturated Fat 2 g

Cholesterol 42 mg

Sodium 273 mg

Total Carbohydrate 2 g
  Dietary Fiber 1 g
  Sugars 0 g

Protein 23 g

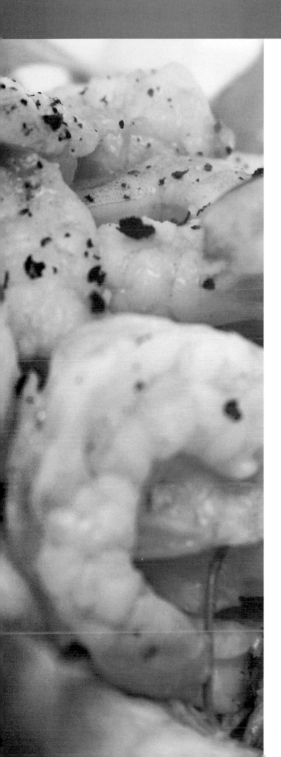

SEAFOOD

SHRIMP AND NOODLES PARMESAN

Serves 4/Serving size: 1 1/2 cups

PREP TIME: 2 MINUTES
COOK TIME: 10 MINUTES

8 ounces uncooked no-yolk egg noodles

1 pound peeled raw shrimp, rinsed and patted dry

1/4 cup reduced-fat margarine (35% vegetable oil)

1/2 teaspoon salt

Black pepper to taste

3 tablespoons grated fresh Parmesan cheese

1 Cook noodles according to package directions, omitting any salt or fat.

2 Meanwhile, place a large nonstick skillet over medium heat until hot. Coat with nonstick cooking spray and sauté the shrimp for 4–5 minutes or until opaque in the center, stirring frequently.

3 Drain the noodles well in a colander and place in a pasta bowl. Add the margarine, shrimp, salt, and pepper and toss gently. Sprinkle evenly with the Parmesan cheese.

COOK'S TIP

If you buy frozen shrimp, place it in a colander and run under cold water until the shrimp are partially thawed, about 1 minute.

EXCHANGES
3 Starch
2 Lean Meat

Calories 354
  Calories from Fat 70

Total Fat 8 g
  Saturated Fat 2 g

Cholesterol 165 mg

Sodium 625 mg

Total Carbohydrate 41 g
  Dietary Fiber 3 g
  Sugars 3 g

Protein 27 g

LEMON-PEPPERED SHRIMP

Serves 4/Serving size: 1/2 cup

PREP TIME: 2 MINUTES
COOK TIME: 7 MINUTES

1 pound peeled raw shrimp, rinsed and patted dry

1 tablespoon salt-free steak seasoning blend

1 teaspoon lemon zest

2–3 tablespoons lemon juice

3 tablespoons reduced-fat margarine (35% vegetable oil)

1/4 teaspoon salt

1 Place a large nonstick skillet over medium heat until hot. Coat the skillet with nonstick cooking spray, add the shrimp, sprinkle evenly with the steak seasoning, and cook 5 minutes or until the shrimp is opaque in the center, stirring frequently.

2 Stir in the lemon zest, juice, margarine, and salt; cook 1 minute.

COOK'S TIP

Serve this in individual au gratin dishes or over steamed rice.

EXCHANGES

2 Lean Meat

Calories 118
  Calories from Fat 42

Total Fat 5 g
  Saturated Fat 1 g

Cholesterol 162 mg

Sodium 327 mg

Total Carbohydrate 1 g
  Dietary Fiber 0 g
  Sugars 0 g

Protein 17 g

TILAPIA WITH CAPER'D SOUR CREAM

Serves 4/Serving size: 1 filet plus 1 tablespoon sour cream

PREP TIME: 6 MINUTES
COOK TIME: 6 MINUTES

1 tablespoon capers, drained

1/4 teaspoon salt (divided use)

1/4 cup reduced-fat sour cream

4 4-ounce tilapia filets, rinsed and patted dry

1/4 teaspoon black pepper

1 medium lemon, quartered

1 Mash the capers with a fork or the back of a spoon. Stir the capers and 1/8 teaspoon salt into the sour cream.

2 Place a large nonstick skillet over medium heat until hot. Coat the skillet with nonstick cooking spray. Sprinkle one side of each filet evenly with the black pepper and 1/8 teaspoon salt. Cook 3 minutes, then turn and cook 2–3 minutes longer or until the fish is opaque in the center.

3 Place the filets on a serving platter, squeeze lemon juice evenly over all, and top each filet with 1 tablespoon sour cream.

COOK'S TIP

Mash the capers extremely well for peak flavors.

EXCHANGES
3 Lean Meat

Calories 135
   Calories from Fat 35
Total Fat 4 g
   Saturated Fat 2 g
Cholesterol 82 mg
Sodium 260 mg
Total Carbohydrate 2 g
   Dietary Fiber 0 g
   Sugars 1 g
Protein 23 g

The filets are cooked
on a broiler rack to
keep any excess liquid
from seeping into the
tomatoes and making
them too watery. The
tomatoes cook just fine
on top of the fish!

EXCHANGES

1 Vegetable
3 Lean Meat

Calories 163
   Calories from Fat 46

Total Fat 5 g
   Saturated Fat 2 g

Cholesterol 76 mg

Sodium 382 mg

Total Carbohydrate 6 g
   Dietary Fiber 2 g
   Sugars 4 g

Protein 23 g

TWO-SAUCE CAJUN FISH

Serves 4/Serving size: 1 filet

PREP TIME: 10 MINUTES
COOK TIME: 12–15 MINUTES

4 4-ounce tilapia filets (or any mild, lean white fish filets),
rinsed and patted dry

1/2 teaspoon seafood seasoning

14.5-ounce can stewed tomatoes with Cajun seasonings,
well drained

2 tablespoons reduced-fat margarine (35% vegetable oil)

2 tablespoons chopped fresh parsley (optional)

1 Preheat the oven to 400 degrees.

2 Coat a broiler rack and pan with nonstick cooking spray,
arrange the fish filets on the rack about 2 inches apart,
and sprinkle them evenly with the seafood seasoning.

3 Place the tomatoes in a blender and puree until just
smooth. Set aside 1/4 cup of the mixture in a small
glass bowl.

4 Spoon the remaining tomatoes evenly over the top of
each filet and bake 12–15 minutes or until the filets are
opaque in the center.

5 Meanwhile, add the margarine to the reserved 1/4 cup
tomato mixture and microwave on HIGH 20 seconds or
until the mixture is just melted. Stir to blend well.

6 Place the filets on a serving platter, spoon the tomato-
margarine mixture over the center of each filet, and
sprinkle each lightly with parsley, if desired.

NO-FRY FISH FRY

Serves 4/Serving size: 1 filet

PREP TIME: 7 MINUTES
COOK TIME: 6 MINUTES

2 tablespoons yellow cornmeal

2 teaspoons Cajun seasoning

4 4-ounce tilapia filets (or any mild, lean white fish filets), rinsed and patted dry

1/8 teaspoon salt

Lemon wedges (optional)

1   Preheat the broiler.

2   Coat a broiler rack and pan with nonstick cooking spray and set aside.

3   Mix the cornmeal and Cajun seasoning thoroughly in a shallow pan, such as a pie plate. Coat each filet with nonstick cooking spray and coat evenly with the cornmeal mixture.

4   Place the filets on the rack and broil 6 inches away from the heat source for 3 minutes on each side.

5   Place the filets on a serving platter, sprinkle each evenly with salt, and serve with lemon wedges, if desired.

COOK'S TIP

Serve this dish immediately after you prepare it for peak flavor and texture.

EXCHANGES

1/2 Starch
2 Lean Meat

Calories 134
    Calories from Fat 23

Total Fat 3 g
    Saturated Fat 1 g

Cholesterol 76 mg

Sodium 239 mg

Total Carbohydrate 5 g
    Dietary Fiber 0 g
    Sugars 0 g

Protein 23 g

COOK'S TIP

Lining the baking sheet with foil makes for an easy clean-up!

EXCHANGES

3 Lean Meat

Calories 156
  Calories from Fat 32

Total Fat 4 g
  Saturated Fat 2 g

Cholesterol 46 mg

Sodium 540 mg

Total Carbohydrate 3 g
  Dietary Fiber 1 g
  Sugars 2 g

Protein 27 g

RED SNAPPER WITH FRESH TOMATO-BASIL SAUCE

Serves 4/Serving size: 1 filet plus 1/2 cup sauce

PREP TIME: 8 MINUTES
COOK TIME: 12–15 MINUTES

4 4-ounce snapper filets (or any mild, lean white fish filets), rinsed and patted dry

1/2 teaspoon salt (divided use)

1/8 teaspoon black pepper

1 pint grape tomatoes, quartered (2 cups total)

2 tablespoons chopped fresh basil

2 ounces crumbled, reduced-fat, sun-dried tomato and basil feta cheese

1 Preheat the oven to 400 degrees.

2 Line a baking sheet with foil and coat with nonstick cooking spray. Arrange the filets on the foil about 2 inches apart. Sprinkle them evenly with 1/4 teaspoon salt and the pepper. Bake 12–15 minutes or until the filets are opaque in the center.

3 Combine the tomatoes, basil, and 1/4 teaspoon salt in a small saucepan. Cook over medium-high heat for 2 minutes or until the tomatoes are limp.

4 Place the filets on a serving platter, spoon the tomatoes evenly over the filets, and sprinkle each with feta.

FLOUNDER WITH ZESTY CUCUMBER TOPPING

Serves 4/Serving size: 1 filet plus 1 1/2 tablespoons sauce

PREP TIME: 7 MINUTES
COOK TIME: 12–15 MINUTES

4 4-ounce flounder filets (or any mild, lean white fish filets), rinsed and patted dry

1/4 teaspoon black pepper

1/2 medium cucumber, peeled, seeded, and finely chopped

2 tablespoons reduced-fat mayonnaise

1/2 teaspoon lime zest

1 tablespoon lime juice

1/4 teaspoon salt

Lime wedges (optional)

1. Preheat the oven to 400 degrees.

2. Line a baking sheet with foil and coat with nonstick cooking spray. Arrange the filets on the foil about 2 inches apart. Coat the filets with nonstick cooking spray, sprinkle them evenly with pepper, and bake 12–15 minutes or until the filets are opaque in the center.

3. Meanwhile, stir the mayonnaise, lime zest, juice, and salt together in a small bowl until well blended.

4. Place the filets on a serving platter, spoon sauce over the center of each, and serve with extra lime wedges alongside, if desired.

COOK'S TIP

Coating the filets with nonstick cooking spray keeps them moist while baking—without many calories from extra oil!

EXCHANGES

3 Lean Meat

Calories 130
  Calories from Fat 33

Total Fat 4 g
  Saturated Fat 1 g

Cholesterol 62 mg

Sodium 299 mg

Total Carbohydrate 1 g
  Dietary Fiber 0 g
  Sugars 1 g

Protein 22 g

SHRIMP AND SAUSAGE RICE

Serves 4/Serving size: 1 cup

PREP TIME: 10 MINUTES
COOK TIME: 23 MINUTES
STAND TIME: 5 MINUTES

4 ounces 50% reduced-fat pork breakfast sausage

16 ounces frozen pepper stir-fry, thawed

1 1/4 cups water

3/4 cup instant brown rice

12 ounces peeled raw shrimp, rinsed and patted dry

1/2 teaspoon salt

1/4 teaspoon black pepper

1 Place a large nonstick skillet over medium-high heat until hot. Coat the skillet with nonstick cooking spray, add the sausage, and cook until browned, breaking up large pieces while cooking. Set the sausage aside to drain on paper towels.

2 Recoat the skillet with nonstick cooking spray, add the pepper stir-fry mixture, increase the heat to high, and cook 3 minutes or until most of the liquid has evaporated.

3 Add the water and bring to a boil. Reduce the heat, cover tightly, and simmer 10 minutes or until vegetables are tender. Add the rice and shrimp, cover, and cook 5 minutes.

4 Remove from the heat and stir in the sausage, salt, and pepper. Cover tightly and let stand 5 minutes or until the liquid is absorbed.

COOK'S TIP

The sausage is added at the very end of the cooking process for enhanced flavor.

EXCHANGES

1 1/2 Starch
1 Vegetable
2 Lean Meat

Calories 269
 Calories from Fat 68

Total Fat 8 g
 Saturated Fat 2 g

Cholesterol 140 mg

Sodium 615 mg

Total Carbohydrate 29 g
 Dietary Fiber 3 g
 Sugars 4 g

Protein 21 g

TUNA STEAKS WITH GARLIC AIOLI

Serves 4/Serving size: 1 steak plus 2 tablespoons sauce

PREP TIME: 5 MINUTES
COOK TIME: 6 MINUTES

1/4 cup reduced-fat mayonnaise

1/4 cup fat-free sour cream

1/2 teaspoon minced garlic

1/2 teaspoon salt (divided use)

1/4 teaspoon black pepper

4 4-ounce tuna steaks, rinsed and patted dry

1   Preheat the grill over high heat, or preheat the broiler.

2   Stir the mayonnaise, sour cream, garlic, and 1/4 teaspoon salt together in a small bowl and set aside.

3   Sprinkle 1/4 teaspoon salt and the pepper over the steaks. Coat the grill or broiler rack and pan with nonstick cooking spray. Grill or broil the steaks 3 minutes on each side or until they are done as desired.

4   Serve the sauce alongside the steaks.

COOK'S TIP

Fresh tuna should be grilled very lightly, so that it's still very pink in the center, for peak flavor and texture. Be careful not to overcook it—the tuna dries out and loses flavor very quickly.

EXCHANGES

4 Lean Meat

Calories 218
  Calories from Fat 93

Total Fat 10 g
  Saturated Fat 2 g

Cholesterol 47 mg

Sodium 470 mg

Total Carbohydrate 2 g
  Dietary Fiber 0 g
  Sugars 1 g

Protein 27 g

COOK'S TIP

Using the lemon slices as a "bed" for the salmon to cook on not only prevents the delicate fish from sticking to the foil, but allows the oils from the lemon rind to penetrate into the salmon, giving it great lemony flavor.

EXCHANGES

3 Lean Meat
1 Fat

Calories 195
  Calories from Fat 88

Tolul Fat 10 g
  Saturated Fat 2 g

Cholesterol 77 mg

Sodium 207 mg

Total Carbohydrate 1 g
  Dietary Fiber 0 g
  Sugars 0 g

Protein 24 g

SALMON WITH LEMON-THYME SLICES

Serves 4/Serving size: 1 filet

PREP TIME: 5 MINUTES
COOK TIME: 10–12 MINUTES

2 medium lemons

4 4-ounce salmon filets, rinsed and patted dry, skinned (if desired)

1/2 teaspoon dried thyme, crushed

1/4 teaspoon salt

1/4 teaspoon black pepper

1 Preheat the oven to 400 degrees.

2 Line a baking sheet with foil and coat with nonstick cooking spray. Slice one of the lemons into 8 rounds and arrange on the baking sheet.

3 Place the salmon on top of the lemon slices, spray the salmon lightly with nonstick cooking spray, and sprinkle evenly with the thyme, salt, and pepper. Bake the salmon 10–12 minutes or until it flakes with a fork.

4 Cut the other lemon in quarters and squeeze lemon juice evenly over all.

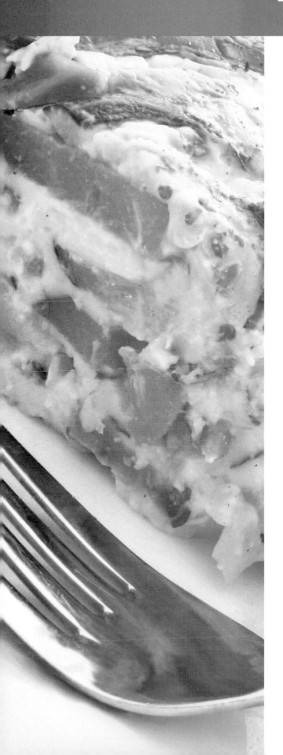

VEGETARIAN DISHES

SPEEDY GREEK ORZO SALAD

Serves 9/Serving size: 1/2 cup

PREP TIME: 4 MINUTES
COOK TIME: 7 MINUTES
CHILL TIME: 1 HOUR

8 ounces uncooked orzo pasta

1/2 cup reduced-fat olive oil vinaigrette salad dressing
(divided use)

3 tablespoons Greek seasoning (sold in jars in the spice aisle)

4 ounces crumbled, reduced-fat, sun-dried tomato and basil feta
cheese

2 tablespoons chopped fresh parsley (optional)

1 Cook the pasta according to package directions, omitting any salt and fat.

2 Meanwhile, stir 1/4 cup salad dressing and the Greek seasoning together in a medium bowl.

3 Drain the pasta in a colander and run under cold water until cooled. Shake off excess liquid and add it to the salad dressing mixture. Toss well, then add the feta and toss gently. Cover the bowl with plastic wrap and refrigerate at least 1 hour.

4 At serving time, add 1/4 cup salad dressing and toss to coat. Sprinkle with parsley, if desired.

COOK'S TIP

Greek seasoning in jars contains dried oregano, mint, garlic, and other herbs. Don't confuse it with the Greek seasoning blend that contains salt.

EXCHANGES

1 1/2 Starch
1/2 Fat

Calories 135
  Calories from Fat 36

Total Fat 4 g
  Saturated Fat 1 g

Cholesterol 4 mg

Sodium 304 mg

Total Carbohydrate 19 g
  Dietary Fiber 1 g
  Sugars 3 g

Protein 6 g

COOK'S TIP

Evaporated milk gives a creamier, deeper flavor than other milk varieties—try it whenever you want an especially rich dish.

EXCHANGES

3 Starch
1/2 Fat

Calories 270
  Calories from Fat 40

Total Fat 4 g
  Saturated Fat 2 g

Cholesterol 8 mg

Sodium 428 mg

Total Carbohydrate 43 g
  Dietary Fiber 3 g
  Sugars 5 g

Protein 13 g

LIGHT PARMESAN PASTA

Serves 4/Serving size: 1 cup

PREP TIME: 5 MINUTES
COOK TIME: 8 MINUTES

8 ounces uncooked no-yolk egg noodles

1/4–1/3 cup fat-free evaporated milk

6 tablespoons grated Parmesan cheese (divided use)

1 tablespoon reduced-fat margarine (35% vegetable oil)

1/2 teaspoon salt

1/4 teaspoon black pepper

1 Cook the pasta according to package directions, omitting any salt or fat.

2 Drain the pasta well and place it in a medium bowl. Add the remaining ingredients except 1 tablespoon Parmesan cheese. Toss to blend, then sprinkle with 1 tablespoon Parmesan on top.

"REFRIED" BEAN AND RICE CASSEROLE

Serves 4/Serving size: 1 cup

PREP TIME: 10 MINUTES
COOK TIME: 15 MINUTES

3 cups cooked brown rice (omit added salt or fat)

15.5-ounce can dark red kidney beans, rinsed and drained

1/2 cup picante sauce

1/4 cup water

1/2 cup shredded, reduced-fat, sharp cheddar cheese

1 Preheat the oven to 350 degrees.

2 Coat an 8-inch-square baking pan with nonstick cooking spray. Place the rice in the pan and set aside.

3 Add the beans, picante sauce, and water to a blender and blend until pureed, scraping the sides of the blender frequently.

4 Spread the bean mixture evenly over the rice and sprinkle with cheese. Bake, uncovered, for 15 minutes or until thoroughly heated.

COOK'S TIP

The refried bean, picante sauce, and water mixture makes a great fat-free bean dip, too! Try topping with reduced-fat, shredded cheddar cheese and serve with warm tortilla chips.

EXCHANGES
3 1/2 Starch
1 Lean Meat

Calories 307
    Calories from Fat 43

Total Fat 5 g
    Saturated Fat 2 g

Cholesterol 10 mg

Sodium 499 mg

Total Carbohydrate 53 g
    Dietary Fiber 8 g
    Sugars 3 g

Protein 14 g

CHEESY TORTILLA ROUNDS

Serves 4/Serving size: 1 tortilla round

PREP TIME: 15 MINUTES
COOK TIME: 14 MINUTES

4 soft corn tortillas

1 cup fat-free refried beans

1/2 cup shredded, reduced-fat mozzarella cheese

1 poblano chili pepper, seeded and thinly sliced,
or 2 jalapeño chili peppers, seeded and thinly sliced

Lime wedges (optional)

1 Preheat the broiler.

2 Place a large nonstick skillet over medium-high heat until hot. Coat the skillet with nonstick cooking spray. Place two tortillas in the skillet and cook 1 minute or until they begin to lightly brown on the bottom. Turn them and cook 1 minute, then place on a baking sheet. Repeat with the other two tortillas.

3 Return the skillet to medium-high heat, coat with nonstick cooking spray, and add the peppers. Coat the peppers with nonstick cooking spray and cook 6 minutes or until they are tender and brown, stirring frequently. Remove them from the heat.

4 Spread equal amounts of beans evenly on each tortilla. Broil 4 inches away from the heat source for 1 minute. Sprinkle the cheese and pepper slices evenly over each tortilla and broil another 2 minutes or until the cheese has melted. Serve with lime wedges, if desired.

COOK'S TIP

For a spicier dish, use seeded jalapeños rather than the milder poblano peppers.

EXCHANGES

1 1/2 Starch
1 Lean Meat

Calories 157
   Calories from Fat 24

Total Fat 3 g
   Saturated Fat 1 g

Cholesterol 8 mg

Sodium 414 mg

Total Carbohydrate 24 g
   Dietary Fiber 6 g
   Sugars 2 g

Protein 9 g

COUNTRY VEGETABLE AND THYME QUICHE

Serves 4/Serving size: 1/4 recipe

PREP TIME: 5 MINUTES
COOK TIME: 35 MINUTES
STAND TIME: 10 MINUTES

1 pound frozen corn and vegetable blend
(or your favorite vegetable blend), thawed

1/2 teaspoon dried thyme

1/4 teaspoon salt

1/4 teaspoon black pepper

1 1/2 cups egg substitute

1/2 cup shredded, reduced-fat, sharp cheddar cheese

1 Preheat the oven to 350 degrees.

2 Coat a 9-inch deep-dish pie pan with nonstick cooking
spray. Place the vegetables in the pan and sprinkle them
evenly with thyme, salt, and pepper. Pour egg substitute
over the vegetables and bake 35 minutes or until just set.

3 Remove the quiche from the oven, sprinkle evenly with
the cheese, and let stand 10 minutes to melt the cheese
and let the quiche set.

COOK'S TIP

To thaw frozen
vegetables quickly, place
them in a colander and
run under cold water
for 20–30 seconds.
Shake off any excess
liquid before adding
them to the pie pan.

EXCHANGES

1 Starch
2 Lean Meat

Calories 153
    Calories from Fat 29

Total Fat 3 g
    Saturated Fat 2 g

Cholesterol 10 mg

Sodium 501 mg

Total Carbohydrate 17 g
    Dietary Fiber 3 g
    Sugars 5 g

Protein 16 g

TOMATO TOPPER OVER ANYTHING

Serves 3/Serving size: 1/2 cup

PREP TIME: 4 MINUTES
COOK TIME: 22 MINUTES
STAND TIME: 5 MINUTES

14.5-ounce can tomatoes with green pepper and onion

1/2 cup chopped roasted red peppers

2–3 tablespoons chopped fresh basil

2 teaspoons extra virgin olive oil

1 Bring the tomatoes and peppers to boil in a medium saucepan. Reduce the heat and simmer, uncovered, for 15 minutes or until slightly thickened, stirring occasionally.

2 Remove the mixture from the heat, stir in the basil and oil, and let stand 5 minutes to develop flavors.

COOK'S TIP

This recipe doubles easily, and is delicious served over whole wheat pasta or steamed veggies (top with a little reduced-fat, shredded cheddar cheese to boost the protein).

EXCHANGES

2 Vegetable
1/2 Fat

Calories 83
  Calories from Fat 28

Total Ful 3 g
  Saturated Fat 0 g

Cholesterol 0 mg

Sodium 609 mg

Total Carbohydrate 12 g
  Dietary Fiber 3 g
  Sugars 9 g

Protein 2 g

BROCCOLI AND TOASTED NUT PILAF

Serves 4/Serving size: 1 1/4 cups

PREP TIME: 5 MINUTES
COOK TIME: 28 MINUTES
STAND TIME: 2–3 MINUTES

1/3 cup pecan pieces

5-ounce package long grain and wild rice with seasonings

2 cups frozen broccoli florets, thawed

2 cups frozen corn kernels, thawed

1/2 cup water

1/4 teaspoon salt

1/8 teaspoon black pepper

1 Place a medium saucepan over medium heat until hot. Add the nuts and cook 2–3 minutes or until they begin to lightly brown and smell fragrant, stirring frequently. Place them on a plate and set aside.

2 Add the amount of water called for on the rice package to the saucepan. Bring to a boil, then add the rice and seasonings. Return to a boil, reduce the heat, cover tightly, and cook 20 minutes. Add the broccoli, corn, and water to the rice and stir. Cover and cook another 5 minutes or until the broccoli is just tender.

3 Remove the rice from the heat and add the pecans, salt, and pepper. Let stand 2–3 minutes if any liquid remains in the pot.

COOK'S TIP

For an even more protein-packed dish, substitute frozen, shelled edamame (green soybeans) for the broccoli.

EXCHANGES
3 Starch
1 Vegetable
1/2 Fat

Calories 275
  Calories from Fat 69
Total Fat 8 g
  Saturated Fat 1 g
Cholesterol 0 mg
Sodium 564 mg
Total Carbohydrate 48 g
  Dietary Fiber 6 g
  Sugars 5 g
Protein 10 g

BLACK BEAN AND CORN BOWL

Serves 4/Serving size: 1 1/4 cups plus 2 tablespoons sour cream

PREP TIME: 4 MINUTES
COOK TIME: 22 MINUTES

10.5-ounce can mild tomatoes with green chilis

15-ounce can black beans, rinsed and drained

2 cups frozen corn kernels

1/2 cup reduced-fat sour cream

1 Place all ingredients except the sour cream in a large saucepan. Bring to a boil over high heat, then reduce the heat, cover, and simmer 20 minutes.

2 Serve in 4 individual bowls topped with 2 tablespoons sour cream.

COOK'S TIP

Don't confuse the 10.5-ounce can of tomatoes with green chilis with the 14.5-ounce can of tomatoes with Mexican seasonings. The smaller can has a bit more spice and a fresher flavor.

EXCHANGES

2 Starch
1 Vegetable
1/2 Fat

Calories 169
   Calories from Fat 29

Total Fat 3 g
   Saturated Fat 2 g

Cholesterol 12 mg

Sodium 415 mg

Total Carbohydrate 35 g
   Dietary Fiber 8 g
   Sugars 7 g

Protein 10 g

SKILLET-GRILLED MEATLESS BURGERS WITH SPICY SOUR CREAM

Serves 4/Serving size: 1 burger

PREP TIME: 8 MINUTES
COOK TIME: 15 MINUTES

4 soy protein burgers (preferably the grilled variety)

1 1/2 cups thinly sliced onions

1/4 teaspoon salt (divided use)

1/4 cup fat-free sour cream

4–6 drops chipotle-flavored hot sauce

1 Place a large nonstick skillet over medium heat until hot. Coat the skillet with nonstick cooking spray, add the patties, and cook 4 minutes on each side. Set the patties aside on a separate plate and cover with foil to keep warm.

2 Coat the skillet with nonstick cooking spray and increase the heat to medium high. Add the onions and 1/8 teaspoon salt. Lightly coat the onions with nonstick cooking spray and cook 5 minutes or until they are richly browned, stirring frequently.

3 Meanwhile, stir the sour cream, hot sauce, and 1/8 teaspoon salt together in a small bowl.

4 When the onions are browned, push them to one side of the skillet and add the patties. Spoon the onions on top of the patties and cook 1–2 minutes longer to heat thoroughly. Top each patty with 1 tablespoon sour cream.

COOK'S TIP

If you can't find chipotle-flavored hot sauce, you can use 1/2 to 3/4 teaspoon of the adobo sauce that is packed with chipotle chili peppers.

EXCHANGES

1/2 Starch
1 Vegetable
2 Lean Meat

Calories 147
    Calories from Fat 32

Total Fat 4 g
    Saturated Fat 1 g

Cholesterol 3 mg

Sodium 525 mg

Total Carbohydrate 13 g
    Dietary Fiber 5 g
    Sugars 3 g

Protein 16 g

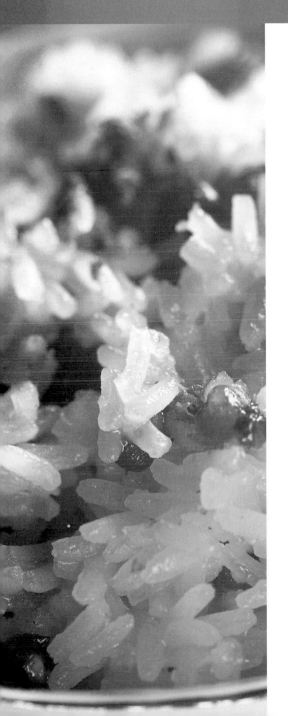

POTATOES, PASTA, AND WHOLE GRAINS

PAPRIKA-ROASTED POTATOES

Serves 4/Serving size: 1/2 cup

PREP TIME: 5 MINUTES
COOK TIME: 20 MINUTES
STAND TIME: 10 MINUTES

12 ounces new potatoes, scrubbed and quartered

1 teaspoon extra virgin olive oil

1/4 teaspoon paprika

1/8 plus 1/4 teaspoon salt (divided use)

1 Preheat the oven to 350 degrees.

2 Arrange the potatoes on a baking pan lined with foil. Drizzle the oil over the potatoes and toss to coat completely. Sprinkle the potatoes with paprika and 1/8 teaspoon salt and bake for 20 minutes, shaking the pan after 10 minutes to stir.

3 Remove the pan from the oven and sprinkle the potatoes with 1/4 teaspoon salt. Wrap the pan tightly with foil and let stand 10 minutes.

COOK'S TIP

Wrapping the potatoes with the foil at the end allows the flavors to develop and keeps the potatoes moist.

EXCHANGES

1 Starch

Calories 81
    Calories from Fat 11

Total Fat 1 g
    Saturated Fat 0 g

Cholesterol 0 mg

Sodium 224 mg

Total Carbohydrate 16 g
    Dietary Fiber 1 g
    Sugars 1 g

Protein 2 g

PARMESAN POTATO BAKE

Serves 6/Serving size: 2/3 cup

PREP TIME: 12 MINUTES
COOK TIME: 1 HOUR
STAND TIME: 10 MINUTES

1 1/2 pounds red potatoes, scrubbed and very thinly sliced

1/2 cup finely chopped onion

3 tablespoons reduced-fat margarine
(35% vegetable oil; divided use)

1/8 teaspoon black pepper (divided use)

3 tablespoons grated Parmesan cheese (divided use)

3/4 teaspoon salt (divided use)

1 Preheat the oven to 375 degrees.

2 Coat a 9-inch deep-dish pie pan with nonstick cooking spray. Put half the potatoes in the pan, then all of the onions, then half of the remaining ingredients. Place the remaining potatoes on top, add the remaining margarine, and sprinkle with the remaining pepper. Cover with foil and bake 45 minutes.

3 Uncover the potatoes and sprinkle with the remaining Parmesan cheese and salt. Bake uncovered for 15 minutes or until the potatoes are tender when pierced with a fork. Let stand 10 minutes to develop flavors.

COOK'S TIP

To slice potatoes easily and quickly, use a food processor with a slicing attachment.

EXCHANGES

1 1/2 Starch
1/2 Fat

Calories 135
  Calories from Fat 32

Total Fat 4 g
  Saturated Fat 1 g

Cholesterol 3 mg

Sodium 360 mg

Total Carbohydrate 23 g
  Dietary Fiber 2 g
  Sugars 2 g

Protein 3 g

CHUNKY POTATO AND ONION MASH

Serves 4/Serving size: 1/2 cup

PREP TIME: 10 MINUTES
COOK TIME: 14 MINUTES

12 ounces red potatoes, scrubbed and diced

1/3–1/2 cup fat-free evaporated milk

1/4 cup minced green onion (white part only)

2 tablespoons reduced-fat margarine (35% vegetable oil)

1/2 teaspoon salt

1/8 teaspoon black pepper

1 Bring water to boil in a large saucepan. Add the potatoes and return to a boil. Reduce the heat, cover tightly, and simmer 12 minutes or until very tender.

2 Drain the potatoes in a colander and return them to the saucepan. Gradually add the milk, stirring with a whisk until blended. Stir in the remaining ingredients.

COOK'S TIP

If you don't have red potatoes, just use un-peeled baking potatoes instead. Leaving the skins on means greater flavor, more fiber, and less work!

EXCHANGES

1 Starch
1/2 Fat

Calories 112
  Calories from Fat 24

Total Fat 3 g
  Saturated Fat 1 g

Cholesterol 1 mg

Sodium 362 mg

Total Carbohydrate 19 g
  Dietary Fiber 2 g
  Sugars 4 g

Protein 3 g

LEMONY BEANS AND POTATOES

Serves 4/Serving size: rounded 3/4 cup

PREP TIME: 10 MINUTES
COOK TIME: 8 MINUTES

8 ounces green beans, trimmed and broken into 2-inch pieces

6 ounces new potatoes, scrubbed and quartered

1 teaspoon lemon zest

1 1/2 tablespoons reduced-fat margarine (35% vegetable oil)

1/2 teaspoon salt

1 Steam the beans and potatoes 7 minutes or until the potatoes are just tender.

2 Place the vegetables in a decorative bowl, add the remaining ingredients, and toss gently. Serve immediately for peak flavor.

COOK'S TIP

This dish also looks great prepared with whole beans— delicious with fresh summer beans.

EXCHANGES

1/2 Starch
1 Vegetable

Calories 69
  Calories from Fat 18

Total Fat 2 g
  Saturated Fat 0 g

Cholesterol 0 mg

Sodium 325 mg

Total Carbohydrate 12 g
  Dietary Fiber 2 g
  Sugars 1 g

Protein 2 g

ROASTED SWEET POTATOES WITH CINNAMON

Serves 4/Serving size: 1/2 cup

PREP TIME: 10 MINUTES
COOK TIME: 15 MINUTES
STAND TIME: 15 MINUTES

1 pound sweet potatoes, peeled and cut into 3/4-inch pieces

1 tablespoon canola oil

2 tablespoons sugar

1 teaspoon ground cinnamon

1/8 teaspoon salt

1   Preheat the oven to 425 degrees.

2   Arrange the potatoes on a baking pan lined with a foil. Drizzle the oil over the potatoes and toss to coat completely. Bake 10 minutes, then shake pan to stir. Bake another 5 minutes or until the potatoes are tender when pierced with a fork.

3   Meanwhile, stir the remaining ingredients together in a small bowl.

4   Remove the pan from the oven and sprinkle the potatoes with the cinnamon mixture. Lift up the ends of the foil and fold them over the potatoes, sealing the ends tightly but not pressing down on the potatoes. Let the potatoes stand 15 minutes to develop flavors and release moisture.

COOK'S TIP

The tiny bit of salt really helps to blend the flavors. This is true in many different dishes.

EXCHANGES

1 1/2 Starch
1/2 Fat

Calories 133
    Calories from Fat 33

Total Fat 4 g
    Saturated Fat 0 g

Cholesterol 0 mg

Sodium 106 mg

Total Carbohydrate 24 g
    Dietary Fiber 3 g
    Sugars 13 g

Protein 2 g

SPEED-DIAL SWEET POTATOES

Serves 4/Serving size: 1/2 potato plus 1 tablespoon honey mixture

PREP TIME: 4 MINUTES
COOK TIME: 7 MINUTES

2 8-ounce sweet potatoes, scrubbed and pierced several times with a fork

3 tablespoons reduced-fat margarine (35% vegetable oil)

1 tablespoon honey

1/4 teaspoon vanilla

1/16 teaspoon salt

1 Microwave the potatoes on HIGH for 7 minutes or until they are tender when pierced with a fork.

2 Meanwhile, stir the remaining ingredients together in a small bowl.

3 Split the potatoes in half lengthwise, fluff with a fork, and drizzle 1 tablespoon of the margarine mixture on each half.

COOK'S TIP

The margarine mixture melts right into the sweet potatoes and looks inviting, with a rich, slightly sweet flavor.

EXCHANGES

2 Starch

Calories 154
  Calories from Fat 36

Total Fat 4 g
  Saturated Fat 1 g

Cholesterol 0 mg

Sodium 112 mg

Total Carbohydrate 28 g
  Dietary Fiber 2 g
  Sugars 10 g

Protein 2 g

BROWN RICE WITH PINE NUTS

Serves 4/Serving size: 1/2 cup

PREP TIME: 6 MINUTES
COOK TIME: 16 MINUTES

3 tablespoons pine nuts

1 cup finely chopped onion

3/4 cup water

1/2 cup instant brown rice

1/2 teaspoon salt

1 Place a medium nonstick skillet over medium-high heat until hot. Add the pine nuts and cook 1–2 minutes or until they begin to lightly brown, stirring constantly. Set them aside on a separate plate.

2 Coat the skillet with nonstick cooking spray and add the onions. Cook for 3–4 minutes or until the onions begin to richly brown, stirring frequently. Set them aside with the pine nuts.

3 Add the water, rice, and salt to the skillet. Bring to a boil over high heat, reduce the heat, cover tightly, and cook 10 minutes or until the water is absorbed.

4 Remove the skillet from the heat and stir in the onions and pine nuts.

COOK'S TIP

Toasting the pine nuts adds just the right degree of nutty flavor to the rice. Be sure to use a dry skillet— no oil needed.

EXCHANGES

1/2 Starch
1 Vegetable
1 Fat

Calories 143
  Calories from Fat 46

Total Fat 5 g
  Saturated Fat 0 g

Cholesterol 0 mg

Sodium 302 mg

Total Carbohydrate 23 g
  Dietary Fiber 2 g
  Sugars 2 g

Protein 3 g

ROSEMARY RICE WITH FRESH SPINACH GREENS

Serves 4/Serving size: 1/2 cup

PREP TIME: 4 MINUTES
COOK TIME: 11 MINUTES

1 1/2 cups water

3/4 cup instant brown rice

1/8–1/4 teaspoon dried rosemary

1 cup packed spinach leaves, coarsely chopped

1 tablespoon reduced-fat margarine (35% vegetable oil)

1/4 teaspoon salt

1 Bring the water and rice to a boil in a medium saucepan. Add the rice and rosemary, reduce the heat, cover tightly, and simmer 10 minutes.

2 Remove the saucepan from the heat and stir in remaining ingredients. Toss gently, yet thoroughly, until the spinach has wilted.

COOK'S TIP

For variation, use spring lettuce mix instead of the spinach. It adds a bit of sophistication as well as great color, texture, and flavor.

EXCHANGES
2 Starch

Calories 137
  Calories from Fat 20

Total Fat 2 g
  Saturated Fat 0 g

Cholesterol 0 mg

Sodium 189 mg

Total Carbohydrate 28 g
  Dietary Fiber 1 g
  Sugars 0 g

Protein 3 g

TACO-SPICED RICE

Serves 4/Serving size: 1/2 cup

PREP TIME: 6 MINUTES
COOK TIME: 11 MINUTES

1 1/4 cups water (divided use)

1/2 cup instant brown rice

1 medium red bell pepper, chopped

1 medium onion, chopped

2 tablespoons taco seasoning (available in packets)

1 tablespoon reduced-fat margarine
(35% vegetable oil; optional)

1 Bring 1 cup water and the rice to boil in a small saucepan, then reduce the heat, cover tightly, and simmer 10 minutes.

2 Meanwhile, place a large nonstick skillet over medium-high heat until hot. Coat the skillet with nonstick cooking spray and add the peppers and onions. Coat the vegetables with nonstick cooking spray and cook 5 minutes or until the vegetables are tender-crisp.

3 In a small bowl, dissolve the taco seasoning in 1/4 cup water. Stir into the rice, add the margarine, and stir until well blended.

COOK'S TIP

You'll find the taco seasoning packets next to the taco shells and salsas in the supermarket. Use just a little to give your dishes Southwestern flavor.

EXCHANGES

1 1/2 Starch
1 Vegetable

Calories 119
    Calories from Fat 8

Total Fat 1 g
    Saturated Fat 0 g

Cholesterol 0 mg

Sodium 270 mg

Total Carbohydrate 26 g
    Dietary Fiber 2 g
    Sugars 4 g

Protein 3 g

PASTA'D MUSHROOMS

Serves 4/Serving size: 1/2 cup

PREP TIME: 5 MINUTES
COOK TIME: 10 MINUTES

2 ounces dry, uncooked, whole wheat spaghetti noodles, broken in thirds

3/4 cup finely chopped onion

8 ounces sliced mushrooms

1/2 teaspoon salt (divided use)

1/8 teaspoon black pepper

2 tablespoons reduced-fat margarine (35% vegetable oil)

1. Cook the pasta according to package directions, omitting any salt or fat.

2. Meanwhile, place a large nonstick skillet over medium-high heat until hot. Coat the skillet with nonstick cooking spray, add the onions, and cook 3 minutes or until the onions begin to brown, stirring frequently.

3. Add the mushrooms, 1/4 teaspoon salt, and the pepper. Coat the mushroom mixture with nonstick cooking spray and cook 5 minutes longer, stirring frequently. Use two utensils to stir as you would when stir-frying.

4. Remove the skillet from the heat, stir in the margarine, and cover to keep warm.

5. Drain the pasta, reserving a little water, and stir the pasta and 1/4 teaspoon salt into the mushroom mixture. If needed, add a little pasta water to moisten.

COOK'S TIP

Using whole wheat pasta is a great way to add fiber and nutrients to your pasta dishes.

EXCHANGES

1/2 Starch
1 Vegetable
1/2 Fat

Calories 102
  Calories from Fat 28
Total Fat 3 g
  Saturated Fat 1 g
Cholesterol 0 mg
Sodium 338 mg
Total Carbohydrate 16 g
  Dietary Fiber 2 g
  Sugars 3 g
Protein 3 g

COUNTRY STUFFED SUMMER SQUASH

Serves 4/Serving size: 1 squash half

PREP TIME: 15 MINUTES
COOK TIME: 35 MINUTES

2 large summer squash, halved lengthwise (12 ounces total; use any variety, such as yellow, scallop, or zucchini)

1 cup chopped red or green bell pepper

1/2 cup water

2 tablespoons reduced-fat margarine (35% vegetable oil)

1 cup dry cornbread stuffing mix

1 Preheat the oven to 350 degrees.

2 Scoop out and coarsely chop the squash pulp.

3 Place a medium nonstick skillet over medium-high heat until hot. Coat the skillet with nonstick cooking spray and add the squash and bell pepper. Cook 4 minutes or until the pepper is tender-crisp, stirring frequently.

4 Remove the skillet from the heat and stir in the water and margarine. Add the stuffing mix and stir gently with a fork. Spoon 1/2 cup stuffing into each squash half. Press down gently so the stuffing will adhere.

5 Recoat the skillet with nonstick cooking spray, arrange the stuffed squash in the skillet, cover tightly, and bake 30 minutes or until the squash is tender when pierced with a fork.

COOK'S TIP

Nonstick skillets will work fine in 350-degree temperatures, even with plastic handles. You may cover the handle with foil, if you like. Or use an 12 × 8-inch glass baking dish.

EXCHANGES

1/2 Starch
1 Vegetable
1/2 Fat

Calories 102
    Calories from Fat 30

Total Fat 3 g
    Saturated Fat 1 g

Cholesterol 0 mg

Sodium 206 mg

Total Carbohydrate 16 g
    Dietary Fiber 2 g
    Sugars 4 g

Protein 3 g

ROASTED CORN AND PEPPERS WITH CUMIN

Serves 4/Serving size: 1/2 cup

PREP TIME: 3 MINUTES
COOK TIME: 11 MINUTES

1 medium red bell pepper, chopped

10 ounces frozen corn kernels

1 tablespoon reduced-fat margarine (35% vegetable oil)

1/2–3/4 teaspoon ground cumin

1/2 teaspoon salt

1/8 teaspoon black pepper

1. Place a large nonstick skillet over medium-high heat until hot. Coat the skillet with nonstick cooking spray and add the bell peppers. Coat the peppers with nonstick cooking spray and cook 7 minutes or until they begin to richly brown, stirring frequently.

2. Add the corn and cook 3 minutes or until the corn just begins to turn light golden in places, stirring occasionally.

3. Remove the skillet from the heat and stir in the remaining ingredients.

COOK'S TIP

You can serve this great side dish next to, or on top of, grilled meats and fish.

EXCHANGES

1 Starch

Calories 79
  Calories from Fat 16

Total Fat 2 g
  Saturated Fat 0 g

Cholesterol 0 mg

Sodium 317 mg

Total Carbohydrate 16 g
  Dietary Fiber 2 g
  Sugars 3 g

Protein 2 g

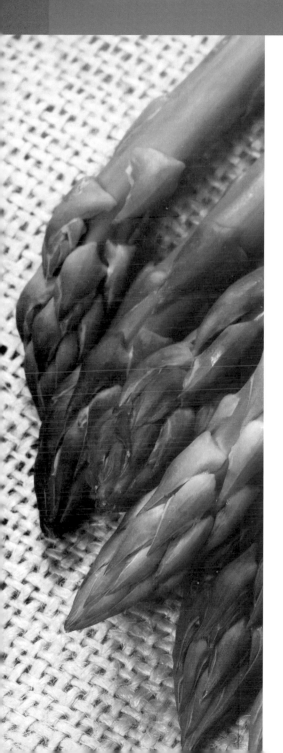

VEGETABLES AND FRUIT SIDES

ROASTED BEANS AND GREEN ONIONS

Serves 4/Serving size: 1/2 cup

PREP TIME: 8 MINUTES
COOK TIME: 11 MINUTES

8 ounces green string beans, trimmed

4 whole green onions, trimmed and cut in fourths
(about 3-inch pieces)

1 1/2 teaspoons extra virgin olive oil

1/4 teaspoon salt

1 Preheat the oven to 425 degrees.

2 Line a baking sheet with foil and coat the foil with
nonstick cooking spray.

3 Toss the beans, onions, and oil together in a medium
bowl. Arrange them in a thin layer on the baking sheet.

4 Bake for 8 minutes and stir gently, using 2 utensils
as you would a stir-fry. Bake another 3–4 minutes
or until the beans begin to brown on the edges and are
tender-crisp.

5 Remove the pan from the oven and sprinkle the beans
with salt.

COOK'S TIP

This side is a great
accompaniment to grilled
meats and fish—perfect
for patio entertaining.

EXCHANGES
1 Vegetable

Calories 37
   Calories from Fat 17

Total Fat 2 g
   Saturated Fat 0 g

Cholesterol 0 mg

Sodium 148 mg

Total Carbohydrate 5 g
   Dietary Fiber 2 g
   Sugars 1 g

Protein 1 g

BROCCOLI PIQUANT

Serves 4/Serving size: 3/4 cup

PREP TIME: 5 MINUTES
COOK TIME: 7 MINUTES

10 ounces fresh broccoli florets

1 tablespoon reduced-fat margarine (35% vegetable oil)

1 teaspoon Worcestershire sauce

1 teaspoon lemon juice

1/4 teaspoon salt

1 Steam the broccoli for 6 minutes or until the broccoli is tender-crisp.

2 Meanwhile, microwave the remaining ingredients in a small glass bowl on HIGH for 15 seconds. Stir until smooth.

3 Place the broccoli on a serving platter and drizzle the sauce evenly over all.

COOK'S TIP

The concentrated flavors in the topping go a long way, so a little is all you need.

EXCHANGES

1 Vegetable

Calories 25
  Calories from Fat 13
Total Fat 1 g
  Saturated Fat 0 g
Cholesterol 0 mg
Sodium 195 mg
Total Carbohydrate 3 g
  Dietary Fiber 1 g
  Sugars 1 g
Protein 1 g

BUTTERY DIJON ASPARAGUS

Serves 4/Serving size: 5 spears

PREP TIME: 5 MINUTES
COOK TIME: 3 MINUTES

1 tablespoon reduced-fat margarine (35% vegetable oil)

1 tablespoon Dijon mustard

1 tablespoon finely chopped fresh parsley

1/8 teaspoon salt

1 cup water

20 asparagus spears, trimmed (about 1 pound)

1 Using a fork, stir the margarine, mustard, parsley, and salt together in a small bowl until well blended.

2 Place the water and asparagus in a large skillet and bring to a boil over high heat. Cover tightly and boil 2–3 minutes or until the asparagus is tender-crisp.

3 Drain the asparagus well and place it on a serving platter. Using the back of a spoon, spread the margarine mixture evenly on the asparagus.

COOK'S TIP

Try this recipe with finely chopped fresh dill instead of parsley.

EXCHANGES

1 Vegetable

Calories 36
  Calories from Fat 15

Total Fat 2 g
  Saturated Fat 0 g

Cholesterol 0 mg

Sodium 197 mg

Total Carbohydrate 4 g
  Dietary Fiber 1 g
  Sugars 2 g

Protein 2 g

SQUASH MELT

Serves 4/Serving size: 1/2 cup

PREP TIME: 5 MINUTES
COOK TIME: 8 MINUTES
STAND TIME: 2 MINUTES

2 medium yellow squash (about 12 ounces total),
cut in 1/8-inch rounds

1 medium green bell pepper, chopped or 1 cup thinly sliced
yellow onion

1/4–1/2 teaspoon dried oregano

1/4 teaspoon salt

1/4 cup shredded, reduced-fat, sharp cheddar cheese

1 Place a medium nonstick skillet over medium-high heat until hot. Coat the skillet with nonstick cooking spray and add all the ingredients except the cheese.

2 Coat the vegetables with nonstick cooking spray and cook 6–7 minutes or until the vegetables are tender, stirring constantly. Use two utensils to stir as you would when stir-frying.

3 Remove the skillet from the heat and sprinkle the vegetables evenly with the cheese. Cover and let stand 2 minutes to melt the cheese.

COOK'S TIP

You need to coat this quantity of vegetables with nonstick cooking spray to prevent them from burning.

EXCHANGES

1 Vegetable
1/2 Fat

Calories 41
   Calories from Fat 15

Total Fat 2 g
   Saturated Fat 1 g

Cholesterol 5 mg

Sodium 206 mg

Total Carbohydrate 5 g
   Dietary Fiber 2 g
   Sugars 3 g

Protein 3 g

MASHED CAULIFLOWER
WITH SOUR CREAM

Serves 4/Serving size: 1/2 cup

PREP TIME: 10 MINUTES
COOK TIME: 10 MINUTES

1 cup water

1 pound fresh or frozen cauliflower florets

1/4 cup fat-free sour cream

2 tablespoons reduced-fat margarine (35% vegetable oil)

1/2 teaspoon salt

1/4 teaspoon black pepper

1 Bring the water to boil in a large saucepan and add the cauliflower. Return to a boil, reduce the heat, cover tightly, and simmer 8 minutes or until tender.

2 Drain the cauliflower well and place it in a blender with the remaining ingredients. Hold the lid down tightly and blend until smooth. You may need to turn off the blender and scrape the mixture off the sides once or twice.

COOK'S TIP

Be sure to hold the blender lid down tightly—the heat of the vegetables may cause it to pop off.

EXCHANGES

1 Vegetable
1/2 Fat

Calories 63
  Calories from Fat 25

Total Fat 3 g
  Saturated Fat 1 g

Cholesterol 1 mg

Sodium 375 mg

Total Carbohydrate 7 g
  Dietary Fiber 3 g
  Sugars 3 g

Protein 3 g

HONEY-BUTTERED ACORN SQUASH

Serves 4/Serving size: 1 squash quarter plus 1 heaping tablespoon honey mixture

PREP TIME: 8 MINUTES
COOK TIME: 7 MINUTES

1 1/2-pound acorn squash, quartered and seeded

1/3 cup water

3 tablespoons reduced-fat margarine (35% vegetable oil)

2 tablespoons honey

1/4 teaspoon ground nutmeg

1/8 teaspoon salt

1. Pierce the outer skin of the squash in several areas with a fork or the tip of a sharp knife.

2. Place the water in a 9-inch glass pie pan and add the squash, cut side up. Cover with plastic wrap and microwave on HIGH for 7 minutes or until the squash is tender when pierced with a fork.

3. Meanwhile, using a fork, stir the remaining ingredients together in a small bowl until well blended.

4. Place the squash on a serving platter and spoon a heaping tablespoon of the honey mixture on the center of each squash quarter.

COOK'S TIP

The heat of the squash will gradually melt the honey mixture.

EXCHANGES

1 Starch
1/2 Carbohydrate
1/2 Fat

Calories 119
  Calories from Fat 35

Total Fat 4 g
  Saturated Fat 1 g

Cholesterol 0 mg

Sodium 144 mg

Total Carbohydrate 22 g
  Dietary Fiber 4 g
  Sugars 13 g

Protein 1 g

SKILLET ROASTED VEGGIES

Serves 4/Serving size: 1/2 cup

PREP TIME: 7 MINUTES
COOK TIME: 6 MINUTES
STAND TIME: 2 MINUTES

5 ounces asparagus spears, trimmed and cut into 2-inch pieces (1 cup total), patted dry

3 ounces sliced portobello mushrooms (1/2 of a 6-ounce package)

1/2 medium red bell pepper, cut in thin strips

1/4 teaspoon salt

1/8 teaspoon black pepper

1. Place a large nonstick skillet over medium-high heat until hot. Coat the skillet with nonstick cooking spray and add the asparagus, mushrooms, and bell pepper. Coat the vegetables with nonstick cooking spray and sprinkle evenly with the salt and black pepper.

2. Cook 5–6 minutes, or until the vegetables begin to richly brown on the edges. Use two utensils to stir as you would when stir-frying.

3. Remove from the heat, cover tightly, and let stand 2 minutes to develop flavors.

COOK'S TIP

Coating the vegetables with nonstick cooking spray helps them to brown without a lot of added fat.

EXCHANGES

1 Vegetable

Calories 17
  Calories from Fat 0
Total Fat 0 g
  Saturated Fat 0 g
Cholesterol 0 mg
Sodium 149 mg
Total Carbohydrate 3 g
  Dietary Fiber 1 g
  Sugars 1 g
Protein 1 g

CREOLE-SIMMERED VEGETABLES

Serves 4/Serving size: 1/2 cup

PREP TIME: 4 MINUTES
COOK TIME: 24 MINUTES

14.5-ounce can stewed tomatoes with Cajun seasonings

2 cups frozen pepper and onion stir-fry

3/4 cup thinly sliced celery

1 tablespoon reduced-fat margarine (35% vegetable oil)

1 Place all the ingredients except the margarine in a medium saucepan and bring to a boil over high heat. Reduce the heat, cover tightly, and simmer 20 minutes or until the onions are very tender.

2 Increase the heat to high and cook 2 minutes, uncovered, to thicken the vegetables slightly. Remove from the heat and stir in the margarine.

COOK'S TIP

For a nice change, serve this as a bedding for grilled chicken or fish.

EXCHANGES

2 Vegetable

Calories 55
  Calories from Fat 14

Total Fat 2 g
  Saturated Fat 0 g

Cholesterol 0 mg

Sodium 266 mg

Total Carbohydrate 9 g
  Dietary Fiber 2 g
  Sugars 6 g

Protein 2 g

SAUCY EGGPLANT AND CAPERS

Serves 4/Serving size: 1/2 cup

PREP TIME: 8 MINUTES
COOK TIME: 21 MINUTES
STAND TIME: 3 MINUTES

10 ounces eggplant, diced (about 2 1/2 cups)

14.5-ounce can stewed tomatoes with Italian seasonings

2 tablespoons chopped fresh basil

2 tablespoons capers, drained

2 teaspoons extra virgin olive oil (optional)

1 Bring the eggplant and tomatoes to boil in a large saucepan over high heat. Reduce the heat, cover tightly, and simmer 20 minutes or until the eggplant is very tender.

2 Remove the saucepan from the heat, stir in the remaining ingredients, and let stand 3 minutes to develop flavors.

COOK'S TIP

Adding the basil and capers at the very end gives these vegetables extra punch, with the flavors "on top" more pronounced.

EXCHANGES

2 Vegetable
1/2 Fat

Calories 72
 Calories from Fat 23

Total Fat 3 g
 Saturated Fat 0 g

Cholesterol 0 mg

Sodium 355 mg

Total Carbohydrate 12 g
 Dietary Fiber 3 g
 Sugars 6 g

Protein 2 g

BUTTERY TARRAGON SUGAR SNAPS

Serves 4/Serving size: 1/2 cup

PREP TIME: 4 MINUTES
COOK TIME: 8 MINUTES

8 ounces sugar snap peas, trimmed

1 1/2 tablespoons reduced-fat margarine (35% vegetable oil)

1 tablespoon chopped fresh parsley

1/2 teaspoon dried tarragon

1/4 teaspoon salt

1 Steam the sugar snaps for 6 minutes or until they are tender-crisp.

2 Place them in a serving bowl, add the remaining ingredients, and toss gently.

COOK'S TIP

Fresh sugar snap peas are available in the spring and fall, but you can find them year-round in the frozen vegetable aisle. They're a delicious cross of sweet peas and snow peas.

EXCHANGES

1 Vegetable
1/2 Fat

Calories 44
 Calories from Fat 18

Total Fat 2 g
 Saturated Fat 0 g

Cholesterol 0 mg

Sodium 184 mg

Total Carbohydrate 5 g
 Dietary Fiber 1 g
 Sugars 2 g

Protein 1 g

GREEN PEA AND RED PEPPER TOSS

Serves 4/Serving size: 1/2 cup

PREP TIME: 4 MINUTES
COOK TIME: 9 MINUTES

4 ounces sliced mushrooms (about 1 1/2 cups)

1 medium red bell pepper, thinly sliced, then cut in 2-inch pieces

1 cup frozen green peas, thawed

2 tablespoons reduced-fat margarine (35% vegetable oil)

1/4 teaspoon salt

1/8 teaspoon black pepper

1. Place a large nonstick skillet over medium-high heat until hot. Coat the skillet with nonstick cooking spray and add the mushrooms. Coat the mushrooms with non-stick cooking spray and cook 4 minutes, stirring frequently. Use two utensils to stir as you would when stir-frying.

2. Add the bell peppers and cook 2 minutes. Add the peas and cook for 1 minute.

3. Remove the skillet from the heat and stir in the remaining ingredients.

COOK'S TIP

Be careful not to overcook the peas—a minute is all they need! Otherwise they lose vibrant color and texture.

EXCHANGES

2 Vegetable
1/2 Fat

Calories 71
 Calories from Fat 26

Total Fat 3 g
 Saturated Fat 1 g

Cholesterol 0 mg

Sodium 225 mg

Total Carbohydrate 9 g
 Dietary Fiber 3 g
 Sugars 4 g

Protein 3 g

HOT SKILLET PINEAPPLE

Serves 4/Serving size: 2 slices

PREP TIME: 3 MINUTES
COOK TIME: 7 MINUTES
STAND TIME: 5 MINUTES

2 tablespoons reduced-fat margarine (35% vegetable oil)

1 tablespoon packed dark brown sugar

1/2 teaspoon ground curry powder

8 slices pineapple packed in juice

1 Place a large nonstick skillet over medium-high heat until hot. Add the margarine, sugar, and curry and bring to a boil. Stir to blend.

2 Arrange the pineapple slices in a single layer in the skillet. Cook 6 minutes until the pineapples are richly golden in color, turning frequently.

3 Arrange the pineapples on a serving platter and let stand 5 minutes to develop flavors and cool slightly. Serve hot or room temperature.

COOK'S TIP

You'll need to buy a 20-ounce can of pineapple for this recipe (or use fresh pineapple slices from the produce aisle). It's delicious served with roasted chicken or pork.

EXCHANGES

1 Carbohydrate

Calories 78
  Calories from Fat 23

Total Fat 3 g
  Saturated Fat 1 g

Cholesterol 0 mg

Sodium 45 mg

Total Carbohydrate 14 g
  Dietary Fiber 1 g
  Sugars 13 g

Protein 0 g

LIGHT GLAZED SKILLET APPLES

Serves 4/Serving size: 1/3 cup

PREP TIME: 5 MINUTES
COOK TIME: 5 MINUTES

1 tablespoon regular margarine

1 1/2 tablespoons sugar

2 cups Granny Smith apple slices

1 Melt the margarine in a large skillet over medium heat, then tilt the skillet to coat the bottom evenly. Sprinkle the sugar evenly over the skillet bottom.

2 Arrange the apples in a single layer on top of the sugar. Cook 1–1 1/2 minutes or until the apples just begin to turn golden. Do not stir.

3 Using two forks or a spoon and a fork for easy handling, turn the apple slices over and cook 1 minute. Continue to cook and turn again until the apples are golden on both sides, about 2 minutes longer.

COOK'S TIP

These are delicious served with pork, chicken, turkey, or ham—or on your brunch table!

EXCHANGES

1 Fruit
1/2 Fat

Calories 77
  Calories from Fat 26

Total Fat 3 g
  Saturated Fat 1 g

Cholesterol 0 mg

Sodium 29 mg

Total Carbohydrate 14 g
  Dietary Fiber 2 g
  Sugars 11 g

Protein 0 g

CRUNCHY PEAR AND CILANTRO RELISH

Serves 4/Serving size: 1/4 cup

PREP TIME: 6 MINUTES

2 firm medium pears, peeled, cored and finely chopped (about 1/4-inch cubes)

3/4 teaspoon lime zest

3 tablespoons lime juice

1 1/2 tablespoons sugar

3 tablespoons chopped cilantro or mint

1 Place all ingredients in a bowl and toss well.

2 Serve immediately for peak flavor and texture.

COOK'S TIP

If you'd like to chop the pears ahead of time, toss them with 1 tablespoon of the lime juice, then cover with plastic wrap and refrigerate up to 2 hours. At serving time, add the remaining ingredients. Try this relish with roasted pork tenderloin or baked ham.

EXCHANGES

1 Fruit

Calories 69
  Calories from Fat 0

Total Fat 0 g
  Saturated Fat 0 g

Cholesterol 0 mg

Sodium 3 mg

Total Carbohydrate 18 g
  Dietary Fiber 3 g
  Sugars 13 g

Protein 0 g

DESSERTS

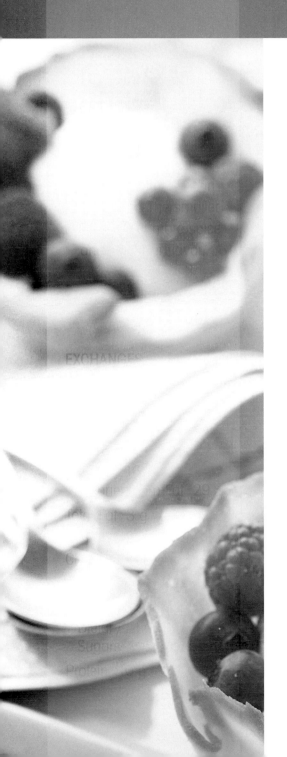

BANANA–PUMPKIN SNACK CAKE

Serves 8/Serving size: 1 piece with 1/2 teaspoon cinnamon sugar

PREP TIME: 5 MINUTES
COOK TIME: 20 MINUTES
COOL TIME: 15 MINUTES

1/2 of a 15-ounce can solid pumpkin, not pumpkin pie mix (about 1 cup)

1/2 cup water

6.4-ounce box banana nut muffin mix

4 teaspoons cinnamon sugar

1. Preheat the oven to 400 degrees.

2. Using a fork, stir the pumpkin and water together in a medium bowl until well blended. Add the muffin mix and stir until just blended (the batter will be lumpy). Do not overmix.

3. Lightly coat an 8 × 8-inch baking pan with nonstick cooking spray and add the batter. Bake 20–22 minutes or until a wooden toothpick comes out almost clean.

4. Place on a wire rack and let the cake cool in the pan for 15 minutes to develop flavors. At serving time, sprinkle 1/2 teaspoon cinnamon sugar over each piece.

COOK'S TIP

For peak flavor, do not top with cinnamon sugar until serving time. You can freeze the remaining pumpkin in a small zippered plastic bag for later use. Store this cake in an airtight container in the refrigerator.

EXCHANGES

1 1/2 Carbohydrate

Calories 111
  Calories from Fat 23

Total Fat 3 g
  Saturated Fat 1 g

Cholesterol 1 mg

Sodium 178 mg

Total Carbohydrate 21 g
  Dietary Fiber 1 g
  Sugars 10 g

Protein 2 g

NUTTY TOFFEE BANANA ICE CREAM PIE

Serves 8/Serving size: 1 piece

PREP TIME: 10 MINUTES
STAND TIME: 10 MINUTES
COOK TIME: 3 MINUTES
FREEZE TIME: 4 HOURS

4 cups fat-free, sugar-free chocolate ice cream

1/2 cup unsalted peanuts or slivered almonds

3-ounce package caramel- or toffee-flavored sugar-free hard candies (26 total)

2 medium bananas, sliced

1. Remove the ice cream from the freezer and let it stand 10–15 minutes to soften slightly.

2. Meanwhile, place a small skillet over medium-high heat until hot. Add the nuts and cook 2 minutes or until they begin to brown and smell fragrant, stirring frequently. Place the nuts on a separate plate and set aside to cool slightly.

3. Place the candies in a small zippered plastic bag and seal tightly. Using a meat mallet or the back of a large spoon, coarsely crush the candies and set aside. Place the nuts in another small zippered plastic bag and coarsely crush them.

4. Spoon the ice cream into a 9-inch deep-dish pie pan, top with sliced bananas, and sprinkle the nuts and candy evenly over all. Cover tightly with foil and freeze until firm or at least 4 hours.

COOK'S TIP

It's best to let this pie stand at room temperature for 10 minutes for easier cutting.

EXCHANGES

3 Carbohydrate

Calories 223
  Calories from Fat 42

Total Fat 5 g
  Saturated Fat 1 g

Cholesterol 4 mg

Sodium 72 mg

Total Carbohydrate 41 g
  Dietary Fiber 5 g
  Sugars 9 g

Protein 6 g

FROZEN CHOCOLATE PEANUT BUTTER LAYERED PIE

Serves 8/Serving size: 1 piece

PREP TIME: 8 MINUTES
FREEZE TIME: ABOUT 4 HOURS

8 chocolate wafer cookies

3 1/2 cups fat-free, vanilla- or chocolate-flavored, frozen yogurt or ice cream (divided use)

1/3 cup reduced-fat creamy peanut butter

2 tablespoons caramel or chocolate syrup

1 Place the cookies in a small zippered plastic bag and seal tightly. Using a meat mallet or the back of a large spoon, coarsely crush the cookies and set aside.

2 Using a fork, stir 1/2 cup frozen yogurt and the peanut butter together in a medium bowl until well blended.

3 Spoon the remaining yogurt evenly into an 8-inch pie pan. Using two spoons, drop even spoonfuls of the peanut butter mixture evenly over the yogurt.

4 Sprinkle the cookie crumbs evenly over all. Drizzle the syrup over the cookie crumbs. Cover tightly with foil and freeze until firm or at least 4 hours.

COOK'S TIP

The yogurt and peanut butter in the second step will be a bit stiff to work with at first, but they will be easier to stir as the yogurt melts slightly.

EXCHANGES

2 Carbohydrate
1 Fat

Calories 194
  Calories from Fat 41
Total Fat 5 g
  Saturated Fat 1 g
Cholesterol 9 mg
Sodium 163 mg
Total Carbohydrate 30 g
  Dietary Fiber 1 g
  Sugars 21 g
Protein 7 g

STICKY CEREAL SQUARES

Serves 9/Serving size: 1 square

PREP TIME: 4 MINUTES
COOK TIME: 10 MINUTES
STAND TIME: 1 HOUR

4 cups whole wheat or corn flake cereal

2 tablespoons regular corn oil margarine

1 cup mini marshmallows

3 tablespoons corn syrup, preferably dark

1 Place the cereal in a large bowl and set aside.

2 Melt the margarine in a medium saucepan over medium heat. Add marshmallows and cook, stirring constantly, until they melt. Add the corn syrup and stir until heated through.

3 Pour the marshmallow mixture over the cereal. Stir gently with a wooden spoon to coat the cereal completely. Place in an 8-inch-square baking pan.

4 Coat one side of a sheet of foil with nonstick cooking spray, place sprayed side down on top of the cereal mixture, and press down firmly to bind the cereal together.

5 Cover with the foil and let stand until firm, about 1 hour. Store leftovers at room temperature in an airtight container.

COOK'S TIP

Reduced-fat margarine doesn't work well in this recipe.

EXCHANGES

1 1/2 Carbohydrate

Calories 106
   Calories from Fat 26
Total Fat 3 g
   Saturated Fat 1 g
Cholesterol 0 mg
Sodium 135 mg
Total Carbohydrate 21 g
   Dietary Fiber 1 g
   Sugars 8 g
Protein 1 g

DELICATE CRESCENT PINEAPPLE CAKE

Serves 20/Serving size: 1 piece

PREP TIME: 10 MINUTES
COOK TIME: 33 MINUTES
COOL TIME: 10 MINUTES
STAND TIME: 4 HOURS FOR PEAK FLAVOR

18.25-ounce box white or French vanilla cake mix

3 large eggs

1 1/3 cups water

6-ounce jar pureed pears (baby food jar)

20-ounce can sliced pineapple packed in juice, each cut in half (reserve juice)

1 Preheat the oven to 350 degrees.

2 Coat a 15 × 10-inch jellyroll pan with nonstick cooking spray and set aside.

3 Place the cake mix, eggs, water, and pears in a medium bowl and mix according to package directions. Pour the batter into the pan.

4 Arrange the pineapple halves in rows of 5 slices across and 4 slices down (creating 20 squares) and bake 33 minutes or until a wooden toothpick comes out clean.

EXCHANGES
2 Carbohydrate

Calories 140
  Calories from Fat 29
Total Fat 3 g
  Saturated Fat 1 g
Cholesterol 32 mg
Sodium 174 mg
Total Carbohydrate 27 g
  Dietary Fiber 1 g
  Sugars 18 g
Protein 2 g

COOK'S TIP

This is a great dessert
to serve with grilled
meat or seafood when
entertaining family and
friends outdoors.

5 Meanwhile, bring the pineapple juice to a boil in a small saucepan and continue boiling 6–7 minutes or until the liquid measures 1/4 cup. Remove the saucepan from the heat and let the juice cool.

6 When the cake has cooled 10 minutes in the pan, lightly brush the pineapple juice evenly over the cake and the pineapple slices. Cool the cake completely on a wire rack. You may serve this cake warm, but its flavors and texture are at their peak if the cake stands 4 hours. Refrigerate up to 48 hours or freeze leftovers double-wrapped with plastic wrap.

BERRY BOWL PIE

Serves 15/Serving size: 1 pie round

PREP TIME: 20 MINUTES
COOK TIME: 4 MINUTES
COOL TIME: 2 HOURS

1 reduced-fat refrigerated pie crust

10-ounce jar raspberry all-fruit spread

2 pounds frozen unsweetened blackberries

4 cups fat-free, sugar-free vanilla ice cream or frozen yogurt

1. Preheat the oven to 475 degrees.

2. Remove the pie crust from the package and let it stand according to package directions. Unroll the pie crust on a cutting board. Using a 3-inch biscuit cutter, cut 10 rounds. Roll the dough into a ball and roll out to a layer the same thickness as the original dough. Cut more rounds. Continue rolling and cutting until you have 15 rounds.

3. Coat a large baking sheet with nonstick cooking spray, arrange the rounds on the baking sheet, and bake 4 minutes or until the rounds are just golden. Remove the baking sheet from the oven and place the rounds on a wire rack to cool completely.

4. Meanwhile, place a large skillet over medium-high heat until hot. Add the fruit spread and stir until melted. Add the blackberries and bring to a boil. Cook 4 minutes or until the berries are softened slightly and heated thoroughly, stirring gently and frequently.

EXCHANGES

2 1/2 Carbohydrate

Calories 184
  Calories from Fat 36

Total Fat 4 g
  Saturated Fat 1 g

Cholesterol 4 mg

Sodium 101 mg

Total Carbohydrate 37 g
  Dietary Fiber 6 g
  Sugars 16 g

Protein 3 g

This is a great recipe
to make ahead of time,
because you can refrig-
erate the berry mixture
up to one week and
store the pie rounds in
an airtight container in
the pantry for a week.
Or you can freeze the
fruit and pie rounds in
separate containers and
thaw before using.

5 Remove the berries from the heat and let them cool completely, about 2 hours at room temperature. This allows the flavors to develop and the mixture to thicken slightly. (You may cover the mixture with plastic wrap and store it in the refrigerator. The mixture will be very thick after it's refrigerated.)

6 At serving time, place one pie round in the bottom of each dessert bowl or ramekin and top with 1/4 cup of the berry mixture. To serve this recipe warm, cover the bowls with plastic wrap and microwave on HIGH for 15–20 seconds. Top each serving with a rounded 1/4 cup of ice cream.

STRAWBERRIES IN DOUBLE-RICH CREAM

Serves 4/Serving size: 3/4 cup

PREP TIME: 10 MINUTES

6-ounce container fat-free vanilla-flavored yogurt

1 1/2 ounces reduced-fat tub-style cream cheese

1 pint fresh strawberries, quartered

1 cup fat-free whipped topping

1 Place the yogurt and cream cheese in a blender and blend until smooth.

2 Pour the mixture into a medium bowl, add the strawberries and whipped topping, and stir gently to blend.

3 Serve immediately or cover with plastic wrap and refrigerate up to 8 hours.

COOK'S TIP

Be sure to use tub-style cream cheese—it has fewer calories and less fat than the block variety.

EXCHANGES

1 Carbohydrate

Calories 92
  Calories from Fat 16

Total Fat 1 g
  Saturated Fat 1 g

Cholesterol 6 mg

Sodium 81 mg

Total Carbohydrate 15 g
  Dietary Fiber 2 g
  Sugars 9 g

Protein 3 g

MINT PATTY ICE CREAM SANDWICHES

Serves 8/Serving size: 1 sandwich

PREP TIME: 12 MINUTES
FREEZE TIME: 1 HOUR

8 small peppermint patties (1/2 ounce each)

16 chocolate wafer cookies

1 cup fat-free, vanilla- or chocolate-flavored, frozen yogurt or ice cream

1 Place the peppermint patties in the freezer for 3 minutes. Remove them from the freezer, unwrap them, and cut each into 8 small pieces.

2 Stir the ice cream and peppermint pieces together in a medium bowl until well blended.

3 Working quickly, spoon 2 tablespoons of the ice cream on the flat side of 8 cookies, then top with the remaining cookies. Press down gently so the cookie tops adhere.

4 Wrap each sandwich in foil and place in the freezer until firm, about 1 hour.

COOK'S TIP

Placing the peppermint patties in the freezer a few minutes makes them easy to cut— and they won't stick to your knife! Store in the freezer up to 1 month.

EXCHANGES

1 1/2 Carbohydrate
1/2 Fat

Calories 134
  Calories from Fat 25

Total Fat 3 g
  Saturated Fat 1 g

Cholesterol 3 mg

Sodium 107 mg

Total Carbohydrate 25 g
  Dietary Fiber 1 g
  Sugars 17 g

Protein 2 g

LEMON CREAM WITH BLUEBERRIES

Serves 6/Serving size: 1/2 cup lemon cream with 1/3 cup blueberries

PREP TIME: 5 MINUTES

8-ounce container fat-free whipped topping

1 cup low-fat vanilla-flavored yogurt

2 teaspoons lemon zest

3 tablespoons lemon juice

1 1/2 cups fresh or frozen unsweetened blueberries, thawed and blotted dry

1 Stir the whipped topping, yogurt, lemon zest, and juice together in a medium bowl.

2 Spoon 1/2 cup of the mixture into individual dessert bowls. Top with 1/3 cup blueberries and serve.

COOK'S TIP

You can also serve this dessert frozen on a hot summer evening.

EXCHANGES

1 1/2 Carbohydrate

Calories 121
  Calories from Fat 7

Total Fat 1 g
  Saturated Fat 0 g

Cholesterol 2 mg

Sodium 47 mg

Total Carbohydrate 24 g
  Dietary Fiber 1 g
  Sugars 14 g

Protein 2 g

OATMEAL COOKIE APPLE BOWLS

Serves 8/Serving size: 1 ramekin

PREP TIME: 8 MINUTES
COOK TIME: 18 MINUTES
STAND TIME: 10 MINUTES

4 cups diced Granny Smith apples (about 4 large apples), peeled (if desired)

3 tablespoons water

2 tablespoons reduced-fat margarine (35% vegetable oil)

1/2 cup golden raisins and dried cherries

3/4 cup dry oatmeal cookie mix

1 Preheat the oven to 400 degrees.

2 Coat 8 6-ounce ramekins with nonstick cooking spray. Place 1/2 cup diced apples in each ramekin and sprinkle water evenly over each ramekin, about 1 teaspoon per ramekin.

3 Melt the margarine in a medium skillet over medium heat, then tilt the skillet to coat the bottom evenly. Remove the skillet from the heat, add the dried fruit, and sprinkle the cookie mix evenly over all. Using a fork, toss very lightly until the mixture just becomes a crumble. Do not overmix.

4 Spoon 2 rounded tablespoons of the mixture over each ramekin and bake 17 minutes, or until the crumble is just lightly golden and the apples are bubbly.

5 Remove the ramekins from the oven and let them stand 10 minutes to develop flavors. Serve warm or at room temperature.

COOK'S TIP

This is delicious topped with a little fat-free vanilla ice cream or frozen yogurt.

EXCHANGES

1 1/2 Carbohydrate

Calories 119
  Calories from Fat 20
Total Fat 2 g
  Saturated Fat 0 g
Cholesterol 0 mg
Sodium 75 mg
Total Carbohydrate 26 g
  Dietary Fiber 2 g
  Sugars 8 g
Protein 1 g

PUMPKIN PIE SNACK CAKE

Serves 8/Serving size: 1 piece

PREP TIME: 8 MINUTES
COOK TIME: 20 MINUTES
COOL TIME: 30 MINUTES

9-ounce box white cake mix

1/2 cup water

1 egg white

2 teaspoons ground cinnamon

1/2 of a 15-ounce can solid pumpkin, not pumpkin pie mix (about 1 cup)

1 Preheat the oven to 350 degrees.

2 Coat an 8-inch-square baking pan with nonstick cooking spray.

3 Add the cake mix, water, egg white, and cinnamon to a medium bowl. Using an electric mixer, beat according to package directions. Add the pumpkin and stir until well blended.

4 Pour the batter into the pan and bake 20 minutes or until a wooden toothpick comes out almost clean.

5 Place the pan on a wire rack to cool completely.

COOK'S TIP

Store this cake in an airtight container in the refrigerator.

EXCHANGES

2 Carbohydrate

Calories 144
   Calories from Fat 26

Total Fat 3 g
   Saturated Fat 1 g

Cholesterol 0 mg

Sodium 221 mg

Total Carbohydrate 28 g
   Dietary Fiber 1 g
   Sugars 15 g

Protein 2 g

COOK'S TIP

The cake continues to cook a little bit while cooling in the pan.

EXCHANGES

2 Carbohydrate

Calories 168
   Calories from Fat 25

Total Fat 3 g
   Saturated Fat 1 g

Cholesterol 40 mg

Sodium 264 mg

Total Carbohydrate 33 g
   Dietary Fiber 1 g
   Sugars 21 g

Protein 3 g

LIGHT RASPBERRY CHOCOLATE CAKE

Serves 16/Serving size: 1 piece

PREP TIME: 10 MINUTES
COOK TIME: 28 MINUTES
COOL TIME: 30 MINUTES

18.2-ounce box Devil's food cake mix with pudding

2/3 cup raspberry all-fruit spread (divided use)

3 large eggs

1   Preheat the oven to 350 degrees.

2   Coat a 13 × 9-inch nonstick baking pan with nonstick cooking spray and set aside.

3   Add the cake mix, water according to package directions, 1/3 cup fruit spread, and eggs to a medium bowl. Using an electric mixer, beat according to package directions.

4   Pour the batter into the pan and bake 28 minutes (or 3 minutes less than directed on the package). Place the pan on a wire rack to cool completely.

5   When the cake has cooled, microwave the remaining 1/3 cup fruit spread on HIGH for 20 seconds or until it's slightly melted. Drizzle the fruit spread evenly over the top of the cake.

POPSICLE FUN POPS

Serves 12/Serving size: 1 pop

PREP TIME: 15 MINUTES
FREEZE TIME: 4 HOURS

1/2 of a 1-pound bag frozen unsweetened strawberries
(about 2 cups)

1 1/2 cups white grape juice

1 cup orange juice concentrate

1 cup diet ginger ale

1 Place all ingredients in a blender and blend until
smooth.

2 Pour 1/3 cup of juice into each of 12 3-ounce paper
cups. Place a popsicle stick in each cup and freeze for
4 hours.

COOK'S TIP

Popsicle sticks are
found in hobby stores,
if your supermarket
doesn't carry them.

EXCHANGES

1 Fruit

Calories 57
   Calories from Fat 0

Total Fat 0 g
   Saturated Fat 0 g

Cholesterol 0 mg

Sodium 7 mg

Total Carbohydrate 14 g
   Dietary Fiber 1 g
   Sugars 13 g

Protein 1 g

BLACK CHERRY–ORANGE ICE

Serves 16/Serving size: 1/2 cup

PREP TIME: 5 MINUTES
FREEZE TIME: 8 HOURS

1 pound frozen unsweetened dark cherries

1 1/2 cups artificially sweetened cranberry juice cocktail

1 tablespoon orange zest

1/2 cup orange juice

1/4 cup sugar

1   Place all ingredients in a blender and blend until smooth. Pour the mixture into an airtight container or a gallon-sized zippered plastic bag (release any excess air). Place in the freezer until firm, about 8 hours.

2   Using a fork, shave the frozen mixture into dessert cups. Or if you've used a zippered plastic bag, take a meat mallet or the bottom of a heavy bottle or can and crush the mixture, then place in cups.

COOK'S TIP

If you're not serving 8 people, you can return the unused portion of this recipe to the freezer.

EXCHANGES

1 Fruit

Calories 51
    Calories from Fat 0
Total Fat 0 g
    Saturated Fat 0 g
Cholesterol 0 mg
Sodium 1 mg
Total Carbohydrate 13 g
    Dietary Fiber 1 g
    Sugars 11 g
Protein 0 g

BERRY–PEACH PARFAIT

Serves 4/Serving size: 1/2 cup

PREP TIME: 7 MINUTES
CHILL TIME: 30 MINUTES

1 cup water

0.3-ounce packet lemon or mixed berry sugar-free gelatin

1 cup frozen unsweetened peach slices

1 cup frozen unsweetened raspberries or blueberries

1/2 cup low-fat vanilla-flavored yogurt

1 Bring the water to boil in a small saucepan over high heat.

2 Pour the dry gelatin into a medium bowl, add boiling water to the gelatin, and stir until completely dissolved.

3 Add the frozen peaches and stir until the mixture is cold. Gently fold in the berries and stir until just blended.

4 In each of 4 parfait glasses, spoon 1/4 cup of the fruited gelatin. Top with 1 tablespoon yogurt. Repeat layers. Chill until firm, about 30 minutes, or cover with plastic wrap and refrigerate up to 24 hours.

COOK'S TIP

You can boil the water in the microwave instead of on the stovetop if you prefer—it takes about 3 minutes on HIGH. Be sure to use a microwave-safe dish or measuring cup.

EXCHANGES

1 Carbohydrate

Calories 75
  Calories from Fat 5

Total Fat 1 g
  Saturated Fat 0 g

Cholesterol 2 mg

Sodium 76 mg

Total Carbohydrate 15 g
  Dietary Fiber 1 g
  Sugars 13 g

Protein 3 g

DOUBLE-QUICK RICE PUDDING

Serves 6/Serving size: 1/2 cup

PREP TIME: 4 MINUTES
COOK TIME: 14 MINUTES
STAND TIME: 5 MINUTES

1 1/2 cups water

1/2 cup instant brown rice

3/4 cup golden raisins or other dried fruit

1 teaspoon ground cinnamon

1/8 teaspoon salt

4 3.5-ounce containers fat-free, ready-to-eat vanilla pudding

1 Bring the water to boil in a medium saucepan over high heat. Add the rice and return to a boil. Reduce the heat, cover tightly, and simmer 12 minutes. (The rice will not have absorbed all the water at this point.)

2 Remove the saucepan from the heat and stir in the dried fruit, cinnamon, and salt. Cover tightly and let stand 5 minutes.

3 Add the pudding and stir until well blended.

COOK'S TIP

Don't omit the small amount of salt in this recipe—it blends the flavors together.

EXCHANGES

2 1/2 Carbohydrate

Calories 166
  Calories from Fat 5

Total Fat 1 g
  Saturated Fat 0 g

Cholesterol 0 mg

Sodium 149 mg

Total Carbohydrate 38 g
  Dietary Fiber 2 g
  Sugars 21 g

Protein 3 g

CREAMY TROPICAL FREEZE

Serves 7/Serving size: 1/2 cup

PREP TIME: 10 MINUTES
FREEZE TIME: 1–4 HOURS

1 1/2 cups fat-free, vanilla-flavored, frozen yogurt

1 pound frozen unsweetened mango or peach slices

1 ripe medium banana

1/4 cup apricot all-fruit spread

1 Place all ingredients in a blender and blend until smooth. Pour the mixture into an airtight container or a gallon-sized zippered plastic bag (release any excess air).

2 Place in the freezer for 1 hour (for a soft-serve consistency) or at least 4 hours (for a firmer dessert).

COOK'S TIP

To soften slightly before serving, place this on the counter at room temperature for 10–15 minutes.

EXCHANGES

1 1/2 Carbohydrate

Calories 105
  Calories from Fat 0

Total Fat 0 g
  Saturated Fat 0 g

Cholesterol 4 mg

Sodium 29 mg

Total Carbohydrate 24 g
  Dietary Fiber 2 g
  Sugars 19 g

Protein 2 g

COOK'S TIP

Lemon curd is sold in major supermarkets in the jelly and jam section.

FRESH BERRY AND CREAM MINI TARTS

Serves 5/Serving size: 3 tarts

PREP TIME: 7 MINUTES

1/3 cup prepared lemon curd or apricot all-fruit spread

2.1-ounce package mini phyllo shells (15 total)

1 cup fat-free whipped topping

1 cup fresh berries, such as blueberries, raspberries, or finely chopped strawberries

1 Place the lemon curd or fruit spread in a small glass bowl and microwave on HIGH for 20 seconds or until it's slightly melted.

2 Stir the mixture until smooth and spoon 1 teaspoon into each shell. Top each with 1 tablespoon whipped topping and 1 tablespoon fruit.

EXCHANGES

1 Carbohydrate

Calories 149
  Calories from Fat 27

Total Fat 3 g
  Saturated Fat 0 g

Cholesterol 0 mg

Sodium 43 mg

Total Carbohydrate 27 g
  Dietary Fiber 1 g
  Sugars 13 g

Protein 2 g

INDEX

Vegetarian Dishes

Other books by the American Diabetes Association

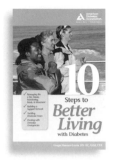

10 Steps to Better Living with Diabetes
by Ginger Kanzer-Lewis, RN, BC, EdM, CDE
Don't let diabetes take control of your life. Instead, take control of your diabetes! Learn the answers to all of your questions about self-care, including the questions you didn't even know to ask. Start living a better life with diabetes— let Ginger Kanzer-Lewis show you how.
Order no. 4882-01; Price $16.95

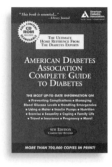

American Diabetes Association Complete Guide to Diabetes, 4TH EDITION
by American Diabetes Association
Have all the tips and information on diabetes that you need close at hand. The world's largest collection of diabetes self-care tips, techniques, and tricks for solving diabetes-related problems is back in its fourth edition, and it's bigger and better than ever before.
Order no. 4809-04; Price $29.95

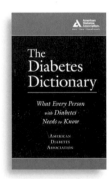

The Diabetes Dictionary
by American Diabetes Association
Diabetes can be a complicated disease; so to stay healthy, you need to understand the constantly growing vocabulary of diabetes research and treatment. *The Diabetes Dictionary* gives you the straightforward definitions of diabetes terms and concepts that you need to successfully manage your disease. With more than 500 entries, this pocket-size book is an indispensable resource for every person with diabetes.
Order no. 5020-01; Price $5.95

Holly Clegg's Trim & Terrific™ Diabetic Cooking
by Holly Clegg
Cookbook author Holly Clegg has teamed up with the American Diabetes Association to create a Trim & Terrific™ cookbook perfect for people with diabetes. With over 250 recipes, this collection is packed with meals that are quick, easy, and delicious. Forget the hassles of meal planning and rediscover the joys of great food!
Order no. 4883-01; Price $18.95

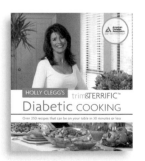

To order these and other great American Diabetes Association titles, call 1-800-232-6733 or visit *http://store.diabetes.org*. American Diabetes Association titles are also available in bookstores nationwide.

About the American Diabetes Association

The American Diabetes Association is the nation's leading voluntary health organization supporting diabetes research, information, and advocacy. Its mission is to prevent and cure diabetes and to improve the lives of all people affected by diabetes. The American Diabetes Association is the leading publisher of comprehensive diabetes information. Its huge library of practical and authoritative books for people with diabetes covers every aspect of self-care—cooking and nutrition, fitness, weight control, medications, complications, emotional issues, and general self-care.

To order American Diabetes Association books: Call 1-800-232-6733 or log on to *http://store.diabetes.org*

To join the American Diabetes Association: Call 1-800-806-7801 or log on to *www.diabetes.org/membership*

For more information about diabetes or ADA programs and services: Call 1-800-342-2383. E-mail: AskADA@diabetes.org or log on to *www.diabetes.org*

To locate an ADA/NCQA Recognized Provider of quality diabetes care in your area: *www.ncqa.org/dprp*

To find an ADA Recognized Education Program in your area: Call 1-800-342-2383. *www.diabetes.org/for-health-professionals-and-scientists/recognition/edrecognition.jsp*

To join the fight to increase funding for diabetes research, end discrimination, and improve insurance coverage: Call 1-800-342-2383. *www.diabetes.org/advocacy-and-legalresources/advocacy.jsp*

To find out how you can get involved with the programs in your community: Call 1-800-342-2383. See below for program Web addresses.

- *American Diabetes Month:* educational activities aimed at those diagnosed with diabetes—month of November. *www.diabetes.org/communityprograms-and-localevents/americandiabetesmonth.jsp*
- *American Diabetes Alert:* annual public awareness campaign to find the undiagnosed—held the fourth Tuesday in March. *www.diabetes.org/communityprograms-and-localevents/americandiabetesalert.jsp*
- *American Diabetes Association Latino Initiative:* diabetes awareness program targeted to the Latino community. *www.diabetes.org/communityprograms-and-localevents/latinos.jsp*
- *African American Program:* diabetes awareness program targeted to the African American community. *www.diabetes.org/communityprograms-and-localevents/africanamericans.jsp*
- *Awakening the Spirit: Pathways to Diabetes Prevention & Control:* diabetes awareness program targeted to the Native American community. *www.diabetes.org/communityprograms-and-localevents/nativeamericans.jsp*

To find out about an important research project regarding type 2 diabetes: *www.diabetes.org/diabetes-research/research-home.jsp*

To obtain information on making a planned gift or charitable bequest: Call 1-888-700-7029. *www.wpg.cc/stl/CDA/homepage/1,1006,509,00.html*

To make a donation or memorial contribution: Call 1-800-342-2383. *www.diabetes.org/support-the-cause/make-a-donation.jsp*